Disability
Definitions, value and identity

Steven D Edwards

Professor
Centre for Philosophy, Humanities and Law in Healthcare
School of Health Science
University of Wales, Swansea

Foreword by

Tim Stainton

Radcliffe Publishing
Oxford • Seattle

Radcliffe Publishing Ltd
18 Marcham Road
Abingdon
Oxon OX14 1AA
United Kingdom

www.radcliffe-oxford.com
Electronic catalogue and worldwide online ordering facility.

British Library Cataloguing in Publication Data

A catalogue record for this book is available from the British Library.

ISBN 1 85775 700 9

Typeset by Acorn Bookwork Ltd, Salisbury, Wiltshire
Printed and bound by TJ International Ltd, Padstow, Cornwall

575752238

Contents

Foreword   v

About the author   vii

Acknowledgements   viii

Introduction   1

Part One   **Defining disablement**   5
                 Introduction   5
                 Why bother defining disability?   7
                 The ICIDH   9
                 The UPIAS definition   19
                 Nordenfelt's theory of disablement   22
                 Harris' definition of disability   30
                 The ICF   32
                 Conclusion   48

Part Two   **Disablement and the idea of a good human life**   51
                 Introduction   51
                 Termination of pregnancy and the idea of a good
                   life   53
                 A hedonistic theory of the good life   59
                 Preference satisfaction as the good life   68
                 An 'objective goods' theory   77
                 A critique of 'maximising' approaches to the
                   question of capacity to lead a good life   87
                 Conclusion   94

Part Three   **Disablement and the person**   97
                 Introduction   97
                 Three philosophical theories of the person, and
                   their implications for disablement   98
                 Persons and human beings   110
                 Disablement and personal identity   113

Narrative identity and disablement   119

Five essential structuring concepts of personal
    existence   123

Disablement and the five structuring concepts   130

The expressivist objection   139

Conclusion   143

Conclusion   145

References   148

Index   153

Foreword

A recent newspaper article reported on a new study that found nearly half of all 'miracle babies' – those born extremely premature, but who were 'saved' by the medical staff – showed signs of mental or physical disabilities by the time they reached school age. The conclusion of one of the researchers was that while he wished they were all 'miracle babies', the reality was 'they're not'. The implication here is that the lives of disabled people are somehow worth less than those without disabilities – for the person, their family, or both.

Professor Edwards tackles this question of the value of disabled person's lives head on by examining three related issues: the definition of disability; the possibility of leading a good life; and the question of personhood and identity. As he points out, these three seemingly disparate issues are in fact closely related; and in this book they are woven together with the idea of narrative identity, which brings a fresh perspective to these well trodden fields.

The great strength of this text is its attention to method and detail. In a field where rhetoric sometimes replaces argument, Professor Edwards is meticulous in presenting a logical sequence of argument and counter argument. In each section he lays out the key theoretical issues, the main contending points of view and methodically refutes or accepts each in turn until he arrives at a well supported and logically coherent conclusion.

A further strength of this book is that Professor Edwards does not reduce his concern down to a single type of disability or impairment. He gives due consideration to a broad range, be they physical, intellectual or sensory disabilities, and deals, where necessary, with any particularities which arise in relation to one or more impairments. This adds a degree of universality to the work, which is seldom found in work in this area.

Though written in the tradition of analytic philosophy, this book has much to contribute to not only philosophy and ethics, but to disability studies, the health and human service professions and, perhaps most importantly, to all of us who struggle with issues such as that reflected in the article noted above. Though philosophically sophisticated, the frequent use of real life examples to illustrate and clarify points under discussion, make it highly accessible to those not familiar with philosophy or academic argument. This, of course, also grounds the book firmly in our everyday experience, which adds to its currency in helping us to engage with complex moral and ethical questions raised by issues such as pre-natal testing for disability related traits.

If we are to grapple fully with questions about disability, then we must look beyond a narrow medical or psychological discourse and examine, as this book does, fundamental questions of what it is to be a person and what constitutes a good human life. Professor Edwards has provided us with an excellent place to engage that struggle.

Tim Stainton
Professor of Disability Theory, Policy and Practice
School of Social Work and Family Studies
University of British Columbia
Vancouver, BC
Canada
January 2005

About the author

Steven D Edwards is Professor in the Centre for Philosophy, Humanities and Law in Healthcare, University of Wales, Swansea. After having trained as a psychiatric nurse in the early 1980s he left nursing to study philosophy as an undergraduate in the Department of Philosophy, University of Manchester. From there he obtained qualifications at the levels of BA(Hons), MPhil and PhD. He has published books on philosophy of mind, relativism, nursing ethics and philosophy of nursing, plus numerous papers in scholarly journals. He is founding co-editor of the journal *Nursing Philosophy* (Blackwell Publishing).

Acknowledgements

Various parts of this work have been presented in various places. I have received helpful comments from many people at such events, in particular, at the Centre for Professional Ethics, University of Keele, at the University of Stirling, and at the University of the West of England. My colleague Hugh Upton was also kind enough to comment on parts of the discussion and I am grateful to him for drawing my attention to the significance of the distinction between 'threshold' and 'maximising' approaches.

Dedicated to my mother EE and to the memory of my father WDE

Introduction

Why a book on disablement from a philosophical perspective? There are at least three main areas of discussion that attract philosophical attention. The first is the extremely fundamental question, 'What *is* disability?'. Perhaps surprisingly there are several differing opinions about this. It will prove important and interesting to examine these opinions and to try to reach a plausible conclusion. Of course certain genetic features of foetuses are routinely screened for prenatally, with a view to establishing a diagnosis of some genetically caused disease or disability. But if there are differing opinions about what disability is, and about the causes of disability, surely this carries implications for the practice of such screening and diagnosis. It may be that we are screening for genetic traits that are mistakenly thought to be disability-causing – i.e. depending upon both the definition of disability which informs such practices, and the view of the causes of disability which informs them. So, since prenatal screening and diagnosis of (supposedly) disability-causing genetic conditions presupposes some definition and some view about the cause of disability, a change in the way either of these issues is viewed will have ramifications for the kinds of genetic traits that are screened for.

To put this point as simply as possible. Suppose we currently screen for genetic trait x and do so because x is thought to be disability-causing. This plainly presupposes some definition of disability. Suppose the definition of disability is revised in such a way that trait x is no longer thought to be disability-causing. Then screening programmes hitherto employed to identify those foetuses at risk of possessing genetic trait x will be abandoned. For if the whole point of screening for x is due to its connection with disability, and if that connection is now severed due to a redefinition of the concept of disability, then the original reason for screening for x is no longer relevant.

It is for these reasons that our discussion will involve an early assessment of rival definitions of disability.

The second main area of discussion centres on the question of what constitutes a good human life. The reason why this is relevant is as

1

follows. As mentioned above, prenatal screening programmes are currently in place. Indeed the UK government is seeking to expand them. And one of the major justifications for the human genome project is that this will generate information that can be used to enhance the current range of prenatal screening tests still further. As is commonly known, screening is often followed by diagnosis. If a genetic trait associated with disability is diagnosed as present within a foetus, very often the mother-to-be opts to terminate the pregnancy (obviously, this claim applies only in countries where termination is legal). This may seem a silly question, but why do people make such decisions? What is the rationale behind them? The proposal to be advanced here is that such decisions presuppose some conception of what is involved in leading a good human life. The presumption seems to be that leading a life with a disability is either (a) incompatible with leading such a life, or (b) impedes the prospects for leading such a life. This presumption needs to be subjected to critical scrutiny. This is done by consideration of some of the main philosophical theories of what counts as a good human life. When this is done, it can be seen that (a) it is almost certainly false, and the extent to which (b) it is true is far less clear than may seem to be the case.

The third part of the book concerns the relationship between disablement and the person. Some see disability as part of a person's identity, in a very strict sense. The 'strictness' appealed to here can be expressed in these terms: the person would literally be a wholly different person were they not disabled. In jargon, such a position is one according to which disabling traits are seen as 'identity-constituting'. This view of disability as something inherent to a person's identity has possibly helped to support the case for 'disability rights', on a par with rights of women or ethnic groups. For the view seems to be, just as being a woman or having a certain ethnic background is part of one's identity in a strict sense, so too is having a disability, or being disabled.

Also, it can seem plausible that disabilities with a genetic cause are identity-constituting. For if any of one's characteristics are part of one's identity, it may be claimed, surely, one's genetic make-up is. However, not all disabilities have a genetic cause. What are we to say in situations where a disability is acquired, so to speak, after conception, either due to injury or disease? Is it still possible in such eventualities to claim that disabling traits are identity constituting? Trying to answer such questions, and to clarify the nature of identity claims involving disabilities will comprise the third area of enquiry to be pursued below.

Finally, it may seem that the three areas of enquiry just summarised are unrelated. But, as will become apparent, there is a unity that can be brought to the three areas in an illuminating way. This unity is generated by the concept of a narrative, specifically of thinking of a human life in terms of a narrative. I'll expand briefly on this claim now. The discussion of definitions of disablement under-taken in Part One will conclude with a view of disability which binds the question of whether or not a person has a disability to that person's own view of the matter. Hence their views on what is impor-tant in their own life will be central to the question of whether or not they have a disability. Such views, as will be seen below, are made against a backdrop of broader judgements concerning what would be involved in leading a good life as far as that individual person is concerned. This in turn will lead us to conceive of human lives in terms of a narrative. So the definition of disability will be shown to be related, at a deeper level, to that of narrative. The same will be claimed in Part Two about decisions to terminate pregnancy when the presence of some allegedly disabling trait is diagnosed within the human foetus. Such decisions presuppose views of a good life for a human being – put another way, of what a good life story is, for a human being. The idea of human life as narrative is expanded and examined most extensively in the third part of the discussion. In this, it will be seen that features of a person that play a central role in their narrative can plausibly be regarded as identity-constituting. Hence, for at least some people with impairments, disability can be an identity-constituting characteristic.

With that brief summary of the contents of the book now completed, we turn to Part One, our discussion of various definitions of disability.

PART ONE

Defining disablement

Introduction

One is presented with something of a paradox when attempting to define disablement or disability. Much work in the area suggests that there is a clearly identifiable group of people who are disabled. Yet, when one attempts to specify just what it is that distinguishes those people who are disabled from the non-disabled, things quickly become very obscure. To see this, consider the following.

Professor Michael Oliver describes himself as 'a disabled sociologist' (Oliver, 1990). The author Jenny Morris describes how she 'developed an identity as a disabled woman, an identity which has been a source of much anger at the prejudice and discrimination that I and other disabled people face' (Morris, 1991, p.1). Being disabled, Lonsdale writes, 'can mean a sense of solidarity with other oppressed people and the emergence of a social and political community of people with disabilities' (Lonsdale, 1990, p.1). Finkelstein points to 'the growth of new organisations of disabled people during the past two decades' (Finkelstein, 1993, p.9). In the same volume there are countless references to 'disabled people' (e.g. p.vi, the contents page), and also to 'disabled students' (ibid.).

In addition it is of course common to hear other expressions that strongly suggest clear demarcations between disabled people on the one hand and, by implication, non-disabled people on the other. One comes across references to deaf people, blind people, intellectually disabled people, and physically disabled people. So it seems as though there is a clearly identifiable category of people who are disabled.

To further complicate matters, it is also often said that were the social environment different in certain respects, then people who currently regard themselves as disabled, would not do so. The claim is that the introduction of changes, such as making public transport accessible for wheelchair users, would have the consequence that many currently disabled people would no longer be disabled. This is a

point of view associated with the so-called 'social model' of disablement according to which the causes of disablement lie in the social
environment, not within the individual (*see* Oliver, 1990 for a
defence of the model).

In virtue of what, then, does a person satisfy the criteria for inclusion in the category of disabled people? The inclusion criteria cannot
require absence of all abilities. Plainly, being categorised as 'disabled'
does not entail that one lacks *any* abilities. At least two of the people
mentioned above identify themselves as disabled and have authored
books. So they have the ability to write books and no doubt have a
myriad of other abilities. Thus being a disabled person need not entail
that one has no abilities.

But there must, presumably, be some characteristic by virtue of
which one is accurately subsumed within that category rather than
the category of non-disabled people.

We've noted the obvious fact that being disabled need not entail
that one possesses no abilities. It is also worth being reminded that
being a non-disabled person need not entail that one is able to
accomplish any possible task or aim. A person may be non-disabled,
yet be unable to write a book. They may have tried but have found
they lack the concentration or sustained effort needed to do so. So,
just as being disabled is compatible with having many abilities, so
being non-disabled is compatible with being unable to manifest many
abilities.

More prosaically, many people wear glasses to aid their sight, yet
they would not typically be said to fall into the category of being a
disabled person. So, being 'non-disabled', or whatever the contrast
class is to 'being disabled', need not entail that one is fully able in all
areas of possible human function or accomplishment. And of course
it is commonly acknowledged that some older people, still categorised
as non-disabled, may have declining physical and mental powers.

Given these points, one wonders what the basis can be, if there is
one, for the distinction between disabled and non-disabled people.
Yet, as Finkelstein's point above asserts, there does seem to be such a
group of people clearly classifiable as disabled. They may identify
themselves as such, and indeed, legislation in both the USA and the
UK suggests as much too (the respective *Americans with Disabilities
Act*, and the *Disability Discrimination Act* in these countries include
definitions of disablement).

Two other features of disablement are also worth drawing attention to. The first is that disablement is a *relational* concept. It is so because it has comparison with others built into it. So to say a person is disabled, or has a disability is to say this in relation to some reference class. The reference class may be other human beings of similar age, and more narrowly still, of similar age within a specific culture.

The second point is controversial, but needs stating. This is that disablement seems to be a concept that is value-laden. It describes conditions that are disvalued. We will be exploring the reasons for this later, but as an indication of the grounds for the claim, the value attached to independence and autonomy motivate the view that disablement is more than just a descriptive concept. For, correctly or incorrectly, it is perceived as being inextricably bound up with compromised autonomy, and with a compromised capacity for independent living.

In this, Part One, of our discussion, we consider, first, why it seems important to try to define disability. Then we consider some of the main definitions of disability that have been proposed over the past 25 years or so. As we will see, all of the definitions have their various strengths and weaknesses. But the theory of disablement proposed by the Swedish philosopher Lennart Nordenfelt is generally endorsed (with some minor qualifications). This will prepare the way for the discussion of the relationship between disablement and ideas concerning a good life in Part Two of the book.

So, let us now address the question of why it may be considered important to define disability.

Why bother defining disability?

We have seen that certain commentators have little difficulty in asserting a distinction between disabled and non-disabled individuals, and indeed that much literature supports the impression that such a distinction can be made. But why might one consider it important to have such a definition?

A first reason, to be returned to later (in Part Two), is this. If a foetus is diagnosed as having genetic characteristics associated with a disabling condition, then it is likely that the foetus will be terminated. Moreover, the UK government and governments in other western democracies, are seeking to expand current prenatal screening programmes (Department of Health, 2003, p.42; Human Genetics Commission, 2004). Since prenatal screening is closely associated with prenatal diagnosis, and eventual termination, terminations of pregnancy on grounds of disabling traits within the foetus are likely to become even more prevalent.[1]

So, being diagnosed as disabled at the foetal stage of development can severely jeopardise the likelihood that one is born. This seems a good reason to enquire into the grounds for the distinction between the disabled and the non-disabled.

Second, if one is born with a disabling trait, until relatively recently, one may have been allowed to die on these grounds alone. 'Allowing to die' here means that nourishment is intentionally withheld from one, or one is deprived of lifesaving medical care (*see* Kuhse and Singer, 1985, pp.3–10). Mason and McCall Smith point out that the law in England and Wales in such cases remained ambiguous up until 1990 (Mason and McCall Smith, 1994, p.153). Of course there is no question of such behaviours being permissible if a neonate displays no signs associated with disability.

Third, it is common to point to the close association between disability and poverty (Union of the Physically Impaired Against Segregation, 1975; Lonsdale, 1990; Oliver, 1990; Morris, 1991; Wendell, 1996). This is due to a number of factors that conspire to obstruct disabled people from obtaining paid employment. Such factors include the poor accessibility of public transport and public buildings, and the attitudes of potential employers, which are prone to be negative and pessimistic about the capabilities of disabled people.

Fourth, being classed as disabled can entitle one to certain social benefits. Thus for many people it is actually important to be classified as disabled in order to claim such benefits successfully (World Health Organization, 1993, p.11).

Fifth, more abstractly, it can be argued that disabled people are accorded a lower level of moral status than that accorded to the non-disabled. To see this, consider that the moral status accorded to a class of individuals is evidenced by the weight of the moral obligations considered due to those individuals. Thus it can be claimed that worms are accorded a lower moral status than humans, since it is considered a much greater wrong to kill a human than it is a worm. Similarly, it is reasonable to claim chickens are accorded a lower

---

[1]For data regarding rates of termination following prenatal diagnosis, *see* www.statistics.gov.uk.

moral status than humans. As with the worms example, it is considered a greater wrong to kill a human than a chicken. And of course, chickens are eaten and battery farmed and humans are not. These points illustrate the way in which the degree of moral status accorded to members of a species (humans, worms, chickens) is evidenced in the ways in which they are typically acted towards.

Consider, then, the following differences in the ways in which disabled individuals are acted towards when compared with the ways in which non-disabled individuals are acted towards.

First, pregnancy may be terminated solely if allegedly disabling traits are diagnosed in the foetus, and is permissible right up until the moment of birth (in the UK, *see Human Fertilisation and Embryology Act*, 1990, sec.37). Hence that is one difference in the ways in which human individuals with allegedly disabling traits are treated when compared to human individuals without such traits ('human individuals' includes foetuses of course). Second, as we heard, until very recently, disabled neonates were legally 'allowed to die' (Kuhse and Singer, 1985). Third, the views of 'personhood' canvassed by contemporary philosophers such as Professor John Harris (1985), among others, lend support to the view that the moral status of humans with intellectual disabilities is less than that of other humans. This is because, in such views moral standing is bound to cognitive capacity. Fourth, the very terminology employed to refer to persons with intellectual disabilities appears to signify a degree of moral status lower than that accorded to other persons – given the high value attached to intellectual *ability* in many cultural contexts (certainly in the UK, USA and other western democracies). All these claims combined lend great weight to the 'low moral status' claim (Edwards, 1997a).

So it is evident that something of great significance hinges upon whether or not one is classed as 'disabled' and so it is pertinent to our enquiry to look now at some of the main ways of defining disability that have emerged over the past 25 years or so.

The International Classification of Impairments, Disabilities and Handicaps (ICIDH) (World Health Organization, 1980)

The intellectual background, so to speak, for this classificatory system stemmed from recognition that many health conditions – illnesses, diseases etc – are not of an 'episodic' or acute nature. They are not of the kind that are manifested and then cured within a short space of time. Some conditions are incurable, some persist as chronic conditions, and some are progressive in character (World Health Organization (WHO), 1993, p.11). The *International Classification of Impairments, Disabilities and Handicaps* (ICIDH) is intended to provide a classificatory schema for such conditions. Not unreasonably, such conditions were understood in terms of their 'disabling' nature, and the general term advocated in the ICIDH to refer to its subject matter is that of 'disablement' (p.1; unless otherwise indicated, references in this section are to the ICIDH). The conditions with which it is concerned are those which it describes as the 'consequences of disease' (p.1).

In the ICIDH it is observed that disease can lead to impairment, which can lead to disability, which can lead to handicap. This is represented in a schema presented thus which illustrates the sense in which impairment, disability and handicap are conceived of as *consequences* of disease:

disease > > impairment > > disability > > handicap (p.11)

Disease is defined in terms of 'etiology > > pathology > > manifestation' (p.10).

To give an example: the cause (aetiology) of a stomach ulcer may be the presence in the stomach of a specific bacterium (*Helicobacter pylori*), the pathology is the erosion of the stomach lining, and the manifestation is the pain or discomfort experienced by the sufferer. To give another example, suppose blindness is caused by a viral infection of the optic nerve. Here the aetiology would be the specific viral infection, the pathology is the damage to the optic nerve, and the manifestation the difficulties in seeing experienced by the sufferer.

Turning now to the other main categories in the ICIDH taxonomy, consider first impairment. This is defined as follows:

Impairment: In the context of health experience, an impairment is any loss or abnormality of psychological, physiological or anatomical structure or function (p.27).

Impairments are said to arise at the level of 'parts of the body' (p.28). To illustrate this, using the two examples given above, the stomach ulcer is actually an impairment since it is an abnormality of anatomical structure (and also an abnormality of function). And it is one arising at the level of a specific body part, the stomach. The damage to the optic nerve in our other example constitutes the impairment in that case. Again this plainly arises at the level of 'body parts' so to speak.

It is worth adding that abnormalities at the genetic level also count as impairments on the ICIDH system (p.27). Thus a chromosomal abnormality associated with Down's syndrome (trisomy 21) counts as an impairment. The relevant 'body part' here is the affected chromosome (even though in effect all body parts are affected since all parts are constituted by cells with this genetic anomaly).

Recall that impairments are said to be consequences of disease, and disabilities consequences of impairments. So consider the definition of disability offered.

> Disability: In the context of health experience, a disability is any restriction or lack (resulting from impairment) of ability to perform an activity in the manner or within the range considered normal for a human being (p.28).

Whereas impairments arise at the level of 'body parts' such as organs, disabilities are said to arise at the level of the individual (p.28). That is to say, impairments are properly attributed to body parts and disabilities are properly attributed to persons.

Returning to our two illustrative examples: Suppose the stomach ulcer is so debilitating that it causes the sufferer to stay in bed, unable to go about her usual activities. That person then has a disability since she is unable to do things which are 'considered normal for a human being' such as venturing outside the home, looking after children, working, pursuing leisure activities and so on. The impairment is the stomach ulcer and the restriction of ability, or the disability, this causes lies in the range of activities the sufferer is able to pursue. With regard to the example of visual impairment, suppose this is so severe as prevent the person from seeing altogether. The person then lacks an ability, the ability to see, which falls within the range of abilities 'considered normal for a human being'; hence that person has a disability. As mentioned, this stems from the impairment which is the faulty optic nerve.

Turn now to the third consequence of disease as presented in the ICIDH, that of handicap.

> Handicap: In the context of health experience, a handicap is a disadvantage for a given individual, resulting from an impairment or a disability, that limits or prevents the fulfilment of a role that is normal (depending on age, sex and cultural factors) for that individual (p.29).

As mentioned, impairments are properly attributed only to body parts, and disabilities only to persons, so it is said that handicap is a 'social phenomenon', for in contrast to the other two consequences of disease this category makes explicit reference to social and cultural factors. (Disabilities make comparison with other humans, but not with reference to specific social or cultural factors.)

Recall our two examples again. First, the 'stomach ulcer' case. Suppose the disabling nature of the condition is accepted, the sufferer finds it almost impossible to get out of bed due to the severe discomfort she endures. This person's disability amounts to a handicap since it prevents her 'fulfilling a role that is normal' relative to persons of the same age, sex and culture. Thus if contemporaries of the ulcer sufferer usually engage in leisure pursuits or work, and the ulcer sufferer is unable to because of her ulcer, she is handicapped according to the above definition.

Consider next the person with a severe visual impairment, so severe they are unable to see at all. It may be said that this person has a handicap by this definition. For, it may be continued, they are disadvantaged, when compared with other individuals from the same culture, of the same age and sex, in fulfilling some specific social role. Thus suppose engaging in paid employment is understood as a normal role. The blind person may be disadvantaged when it comes to seeking and performing this due to their being unable to see. The blindness may limit the range of employment opportunities open to the person. And this may constitute a disadvantage relative to other people in the same culture of the same age and sex.

Again, handicap can be seen as a 'consequence of disease'. In the two examples just considered, the relevant diseases are the stomach ulcer and the lesion in the optic nerve respectively.

It is evident, then, that impairment may be a necessary condition of disability, but is not a sufficient condition. This contingency between impairments and disabilities can be illustrated thus. Conditions such as fused toes or exceptionally large ears may count as impairments. But they fall short of disabilities. Here there are structural abnormalities with no functional consequences. (So impairments differ from diseases.) In the 'exceptionally large ears' example, if the person with these ears suffers from embarrassment about them, they may lead to a handicap, for example if the person finds it impossible to leave her house due to fear of comments about her large ears.

Also there may be provision to mitigate adverse functional consequences of impairments, such as spectacles for the short-sighted, insulin for diabetics. So again here we have impairments but no disability, provided relevant 'external' compensating conditions are present, such as the availability of glasses or insulin.

A distinction between abilities and capacities may be useful here. The short-sighted person has the *capacity* to see, but not the ability. Given suitable visual aids (adequate spectacles), such a person can manifest her capacity and thus attain the ability to see. But the person who lacks an optic nerve lacks both the capacity *and* the ability to see.

It is also possible to point to circumstances in which a disability does not lead to a handicap. In the island known as 'Martha's Vineyard' (Sacks, 1989), a high proportion of the populace were deaf. So all residents of the island were competent in using sign language. The suggestion is that in this context deafness may be a disability but does not lead to a handicap (Sacks, 1989; Oliver, 1990, p.16).

Having set out the ICIDH definitions, let us now consider some criticisms which may be made of them.

Criticisms

The philosopher Professor Lennart Nordenfelt (1983/1997) has levelled three important criticisms at the ICIDH classificatory scheme. First, he points out that although the ICIDH claims to distinguish disease from impairment, these are in fact the same thing. That is, impairments are just diseases, hence they cannot be consequences of disease.

To see this, here is the definition of impairments once again: 'In the context of health experience, an impairment is any loss or abnormality of psychological, physiological or anatomical structure or function' (p.27). This includes the standard way of defining disease within a biomedical model of disease (Boorse, 1975, p.57). In such a model a disease is a condition which impairs species-typical function.

Thus the class of pathological conditions (diseases) actually coincides with the class of impairments, for both are defined in the same manner.

Second, in the ICIDH, intellectual impairments are not properly distinguishable from disabilities. Recall that impairments are said to be properly attributable only to 'body parts' but that disabilities are properly attributable only to persons. But, Nordenfelt (1983/1997) points out, psychological impairments all arise at the level of the person, not at the level of organs or body parts.

Hence, consider an intellectual disability such as lack of short-term memory. One could only attribute this to a person after having seen them manifest this lack. This differs from physical impairments. In these one could diagnose the presence of a physical impairment (such as kidney disease, stomach ulcer, optic nerve degeneration) without observing the person's behaviour. The diagnosis 'lack of short-term memory' would be attributed to the *person*, not to any organ. Of course, this problem of cognition may be a consequence of neurological degeneration. But that degeneration falls under the category of physical disease rather than mental impairment. (Perhaps here the conflation of impairment and disease arises again.) So the class of psychological impairments should be re-classified as intellectual disabilities. As Nordenfelt puts it: 'a disturbance in a mental function is already a disability, therefore there is no need for the category of mental impairment!' (Nordenfelt, 1983, p.27).[2]

Nordenfelt's third criticism concerns the disability/handicap distinction. According to the ICIDH the category of disability is 'value free' while the category of handicap is value laden (p.29). Nordenfelt points out that it is more accurate to state that both categories are value laden. The reason is that the class of disabilities is identified as such because they signify the absence of abilities that humans typically value. (In defence of the authors of the ICIDH it should be pointed out they are aware of the normative nature of the categories of disease and disability (p.33, p.39).)

Of these criticisms, perhaps the first is the most serious for it points to a conflation of two key components of the ICIDH, and if accepted it entails that impairments cannot properly be regarded as 'conse-

---

[2]Though, in defence of the ICIDH, one could say of a person that their memory is faulty – an attribution to a 'part of a person', a mental organ say.

quences of disease' because they are themselves diseases. I suspect that a proponent of the ICIDH could simply accept this, and modify the 'consequences of disease' claim so that it is instead applicable only to disabilities and handicaps. So although Nordenfelt's criticisms are legitimate and important, they still leave the main body of the ICIDH intact in my opinion. They are consistent with acceptance of the four main categories (with the proviso just noted), and with two controversial views: (a) that disabilities and handicaps are consequences of disease and (b) that the disability/handicap distinction is a legitimate one. As we will see now each of these claims has been disputed.

A frequently voiced criticism of the ICIDH is that it presents a view in which the causes of disability and handicap lie in the individual (Oliver, 1990). One can appreciate how a reading of the 'consequence of disease' claim can seem to state such a position, for it suggests that had not the individual succumbed to the disease, they would not have been disabled, nor would they be handicapped.

On a less than careful reading, the ICIDH may seem to say the causes of disability and handicap lie in the individual. In fact the 'arrow' representation used in the text and repeated on p.10 does seem to prompt such an interpretation.

Suppose this interpretation is accepted as a reasonable one. Critics then point out that the causes of disability and handicap lie in the social environment and not within the individual (Oliver, 1990). If all that prevents a person with paraplegia from working is the absence of ramps to public buildings and wheelchair-friendly public transport, then one can see the plausibility of the claim that the cause of handicap lies in the social environment, not in the individual.

The view that the causes of disability and handicap lie in the individual is said to generate a 'medicalisation' of disability (Oliver, 1990). This has several negative consequences. A first is that it fosters the impression that disability and handicap are inevitably accompanied by illness. In response to this it is pointed out that one can of course be healthy and at the same time disabled. There is no necessary relationship between disability and illness, contrary to the impression fostered by a medicalised view of disability.

A second negative consequence of the medicalisation of disability lies in the response to it. If disability and handicap are considered medical problems of the individual, then the appropriate response to the problems seems to be to focus on that individual. Rather than

modify the social environment, the appropriate response to paraplegia, prompted by medicalisation, is to try to encourage the individual to walk, for example with use of aids such as callipers.

A third consequence is to look to the medical sphere in order to
respond to disability and handicap. Thus people with disabilities were
considered to require care provided by medical and nursing
personnel. Some argue this is highly inappropriate given the contingency of the relationship between disability and illness, and the view
that the social environment causes disability and handicap (*see* e.g.
Oliver, 1990; Swain *et al.*, 1993).

These criticisms are motivated by the model presented on p.10 in
which an arrow leads from disability to impairment to disability and
to handicap (p.11). Some have taken the relationship represented by
the arrow as a simple, necessarily deterministic, causal relationship.

In defence, the 1993 edition of the ICIDH states that the arrow
should be read as meaning 'may lead to' (p.5), thus presenting a
contingent relationship between disease and the subsequent dimensions, and not a necessary one.

It should be acknowledged that the mode of expression, plus the
'arrow' representation within the ICIDH invite the kinds of critical
responses just rehearsed. However, as indicated here, contrary to
what some critics claim, the ICIDH does not in fact express commitment to the kind of simple causal relationship which generates the
medicalisation of disability and handicap. The 'arrow' schema plus
the general language of the ICIDH suggest disease is a necessary
condition of disability and of handicap, hence the claim that these are
both consequences of disease. But the ICIDH does not advance the
further claim that disease is a sufficient condition for the presence of
disability. As pointed out in the ICIDH, a person may have a disease
(or impairment) but have neither a disability nor a handicap. An
example would be a pair of fused toes on an otherwise normally
structured foot.

So, strictly speaking, the position set out in the ICIDH should be
seen as one compatible with the view that the causes of disability and
handicap are two-fold. They stem partly from factors within the body
of the person (diseases, impairments), and partly from external
factors (such as a social environment that is not wheelchair-friendly).

Three other final criticisms concern the view of health within the
ICIDH, the disability/handicap distinction, and the relationship
between disability and identity (p.24, p.28).

First, as mentioned, a biomedical model of disease appears to lie at the basis of the ICIDH. This is important since it purports to provide 'consequences of disease' analysis. One criticism of such a biomedical model of disease is that it defines health in terms of the absence of disease. The presence of disease is then supposed to impact negatively on a person's health. Hence, the complaint that the ICIDH links disability and illness too closely may well be a fair one. For, as we saw, disease is a necessary condition of impairments, disabilities and handicaps. So someone who subscribes to a biomedical model of disease may infer that a person with a disease thereby has an illness. Strictly speaking, such an inference would not be warranted since the presence of disease is not a sufficient condition for the presence of illness. A person may feel well though carry a disease entity such as a virus (e.g. HIV). Nonetheless, a person may – however erroneously – infer that people with disabilities cannot be healthy. They may infer this if they suppose that disabilities are inevitably 'consequences of disease'. However, adoption of a broader definition of disease (a holistic definition, Greaves, (1996)) would entail that one could not legitimately infer absence of health when disease is present. Such a judgement would require some general assessment of the views of the person whose health status is in question.

Relatedly, adoption of a non-biomedical model of disease would entail that judgements about health, illness *and* disablement would be answerable to the person's own judgement on the matter. The ICIDH schema does not seem to embrace any such perspective. On that schema, as one would expect from a position anchored in a biomedical model of disease, the question of whether or not a person is disabled or handicapped can be determined entirely from the third-person perspective. The views of the person concerned are irrelevant and need carry no weight at all in such judgements. This is a criticism which has been voiced by a number of commentators (Oliver, 1990; Swain *et al.*, 1993).

Regarding the disability/handicap distinction, one criticism levelled at this is that it is theoretically superfluous (Edwards, 1997b). To see why one might think this, recall again the kinds of abilities referred to in the definition of disability. As we saw these are very abstract, general classes of abilities such as seeing, hearing, walking and so on. They are abilities one might reasonably describe as species typical, and highly general, that is, independent of specific social contexts.

But, the criticism runs, if one is concerned with the kinds of abilities which are really important to the lives of persons, no reference will be made to these very general kinds of act-types (walking, seeing, hearing etc). More specific act-types will be invoked, which are important to individual people in their day-to-day lives. Thus actions such as shopping, studying, preparing food, raising children, working, and pursuit of leisure activities represent the kinds of actions that are most important to people. Hence, it seems reasonable to point out, it is actions at this more specific level which should be the focus of concern in definitions of disability, and not the highly general act-types which figure in the ICIDH. For abilities such as walking, hearing and seeing do not have *intrinsic* value. They are valuable because they are means to achieving what we really do value: the fulfilment of our ambitions, the pursuit of things which are important to us.

In response to this criticism – that of the theoretical superfluity of the category of disability in the ICIDH – at least two points can be made.

First, from an epidemiological perspective it can be extremely useful to have available information concerning the prevalence of disabilities even at the general level specified in the ICIDH. For if, say, blindness or inability to walk is highly prevalent in one social group but not in another this would plainly constitute important data (*see* Bickenbach *et al.*, 1999 for this response). Hence this is at least one good reason for inclusion of the category of disability in a theoretical analysis of disablement.

A second reason is of course that at the clinical level it can be important to focus on the kinds of disabilities which fall within this category in the ICIDH. This may be for purposes of rehabilitation for example. The point that this may not always be the best response to disability is important. But there may be situations in which a person's ability to walk is recoverable with suitable physiotherapy. Such a person retains the capacity to walk but manifestation of the ability to walk requires therapy. Analysis of disability as classified in the ICIDH identifies this range of data and opens up the possibility of discussion and comparison of different kinds of therapeutic regimes. If this stratum of analysis is omitted, these important data are masked (Nordenfelt, 1997). These two responses seem powerful enough to reject the criticism that the category of disability is superfluous.

The other area of possible criticism of the ICIDH concerns the relationship of disability to identity. As this is a topic to be discussed in depth in Part Three, we will raise it here only to note a tension in the ICIDH in this area. Early on in the ICIDH a distinction between 'being rather than having' is drawn attention to (p.28). This is a distinction between *being* disabled and *having* a disability. In the passage during which this distinction is drawn, preference is expressed towards 'having' since this, in the eyes of the authors of the ICIDH, preserves a certain 'neutrality' (p.28) with regard to the person's potential. The expression 'being', though, as in 'being disabled' is viewed less favourably: 'it is to risk being dismissive and invoking stigma' (p.28).[3]

In spite of expressing a preference for 'having', the ICIDH discussion of disability characterises this as a 'change in ... identity' (p.28; *see also* p.24). So the ICIDH seems to express ambiguity concerning the relationship between disability and identity. On the one hand it seems to favour the 'having' concept, as seen above. But on the other hand, specifically in the discussion of disability, it seems to be claimed that disability is part of a person's very identity, and hence that one can legitimately speak of a person *being* disabled as opposed to simply *having* a disability. Having noted this ambiguity, we will postpone discussion of the relationship between disability and identity until later.

Overall, then, it seems the ICIDH may have received some unfair criticism. But at least two important criticisms of it remain unanswered. The first concerns the conflation of impairments and diseases. The second, more seriously, concerns its theoretical basis in a biomedical model of disease, one that appears to deny any role for the view of the person concerned in the question of whether or not they have a disability or are ill.

For now we turn to discuss a definition of disability produced by the Union of the Physically Impaired Against Segregation (UPIAS; *see* UPIAS, 1975).

The Union of the Physically Impaired Against Segregation (UPIAS) definition

The redefinition of disablement provided by the UPIAS was prompted by alleged inadequacies in the medical manner of viewing disablement (as, according to its critics, is manifested in the ICIDH defini-

---

[3]Interestingly, Oliver expressly voices his preference for 'being' over 'having' (Oliver, 1990, p.xiii).

tion). The UPIAS document sought to shift the conception of disablement from that of a medical concept to a social concept. In so doing it would attempt to dislodge the view that disablement is caused by something internal to the person, as a medical condition would be understood. It would instead seek to replace such a medicalised view of disability, with the view that disability has a social cause. For, in the eyes of UPIAS 'it is society which disables physically impaired people' (UPIAS, 1975, p.3). Moreover, the UPIAS observes that medicalised analyses of disability omit to take into account the views of disabled people (UPIAS, 1975).

The UPIAS definition is extremely brief, and comprises two clauses:

> Impairment: lacking part or all of a limb, or having a defective limb, organ or mechanism of the body.

> Disability: the disadvantage or restriction of activity caused by a contemporary social organisation which takes little or no account of people who have physical impairments and thus excludes them from participation in the mainstream of social activities (Oliver, 1990, p.11; UPIAS, 1975).

The two most striking features of this are the causal claim, and the omission of the category of handicaps. On this last point, it seems plain that the UPIAS is using the term 'disability' in a way that is most closely related to the ICIDH use of the term 'handicap'; both are couched in terms of disadvantage due to social factors for example. So, just to be clear, the ICIDH presents a three-level analysis of the phenomenon of disablement, consisting of impairment, disability, handicap. The UPIAS presents instead a two-level analysis, in terms of impairment and disability. But the UPIAS is using 'disability' in a way that closely approximates 'handicap' in the ICIDH. Thus the level of analysis omitted by the UPIAS but recognised within the ICIDH is that of *disabilities* (where these denote the inability to manifest species typical act-types such as walking, hearing, and seeing).

A criticism of the ICIDH discussed above concerned the alleged theoretical superfluity of the 'disability' level of analysis within the ICIDH. Given that the UPIAS finds no place in its definition for a similar plane of analysis it is reasonable to assume it would agree with the criticism of theoretical superfluity. However, as we saw, the theoretical superfluity objection can be responded to and indeed overcome. Hence, the absence of this level of analysis in the UPIAS definition (a level equivalent to the ICIDH's 'disability') is a severe weakness of the UPIAS's position.

With regard to the causal claim in the UPIAS definition, Oliver describes it as follows. The UPIAS definition 'locates the causes of disability squarely within society and social organisation' (Oliver, 1990, p.11). The UPIAS itself states 'it is society which disables physically impaired people' (UPIAS, 1975, p.3).

In the context of providing some radical opposition to medicalised, overly biological analyses of disablement, the rationale for advancing such a causal claim is understandable. But the claim itself is surely false. Three possible causal claims are identifiable. (a) The first, in line with the UPIAS view, is that the cause of disability (what the ICIDH terms 'handicap') lies in the social context. (b) Second, is that the causes of disability and handicap lie in the individual. (c) A third claim describes a position distinct from either (a) or (b) in which the cause of disability (handicap in the ICIDH's analysis) is two-fold, it is partly caused by the social context, and partly by the presence within an individual of an impairment.

The clear problem with (a) is that it does not serve to indicate the difference between social exclusion on grounds of disability, and social exclusion on other grounds, for example prejudicial exclusion on grounds of race or sex in social institutions. The difference between exclusion on grounds of impairment, and exclusion on grounds of race or sex is that exclusion on the latter grounds does not stem from the presence within an individual of an impairment (or disease). Plainly, being female or being non-white does not amount to having an impairment. So, in locating the cause of disability entirely in the social context, the UPIAS definition fails to acknowledge that the social exclusion referred to in the definition is at least partly a consequence of the presence of an impairment within an individual.

It should be stressed that in advancing this criticism of the UPIAS definition, it is being recognised here that disability, in their sense, has a *two-fold* cause: the impairment and the social context. Changes to the social context, if they are brought about, may ameliorate the disability, and even cause it to evaporate, but the impairment will remain (even though its significance will now be vastly reduced since it will not be accompanied by disability).

Before moving on, it is worth raising one other criticism of the UPIAS definition. In the definition of disability given the emphasis is placed very much upon *physical* impairments and 'mechanisms' (UPIAS, 1975). But of course it can be pointed out that intellectual impairments are not, strictly speaking, physical, even if they result from physical impairments such as degeneration in neuronal tissue. Also, relatedly, one can ask if sensory disabilities are properly characterised as *physical* in nature. Sure enough, their proper function requires the proper function of some underlying physical systems, but are the experiences themselves mental or physical? It is at least reasonable to claim they are mental in nature. If this is so, they seem to fall outside the scope of the UPIAS definition and thus the definition invites the criticism of excluding the range of non-physical disabilities. Finally, it is true that the emphasis placed upon the social environment in the UPIAS definition is a useful counter to overly medicalised accounts of disablement, but the definition seems open to too many serious objections to be accepted as an adequate definition of disablement. In light of that, let us now turn to the theory proposed by Nordenfelt.[4]

Nordenfelt's theory of disablement

The Swedish philosopher Professor Lennart Nordenfelt has set out a theory of disability in several places (Nordenfelt, 1983/1997, 1993a, 1995, 2000, 2001). Moreover, the theory has developed in tandem with Professor Nordenfelt's theory of health (see especially his 1995 and 2001 publications).

In a nutshell, his theory is that one is disabled when one is unable to do things which are important to one. In disablement this inability stems from a combination of internal factors (such as impairments) and external factors (such as wheelchair-unfriendly public transportation systems).

In setting out his theory, Nordenfelt introduces the idea of a non-ability. This is the class of abilities which an individual lacks. Hence if

---

[4]The UPIAS definition raises the contrast between two models of disability: Oliver expresses the distinction between these two models as follows: '[The] individual model of disability ... locates the "problem" of disability within the individual and secondly it sees the causes of this problem as stemming from the functional limitations ... which are assumed to arise from disability' ... '[According to the] social model it is not individual limitations ... which are the cause of the problem but society's failure to provide appropriate services and adequately ensure the needs of disabled people are fully taken into account in its social organisation' (Oliver, 1990, p.32).

one cannot play chess, then one has a non-ability to play chess. Obviously not all non-abilities constitute disabilities. Those non-abilities that constitute disabilities stem at least partly from factors intrinsic to the individual. Thus 'disability, in contradistinction to ... non-ability, is tied to those conditions which are *inherent* in the agent himself' (Nordenfelt, 1983, p.51). So in terminology familiar from the ICIDH, we may say that disabilities are non-abilities which stem from the presence of some impairment in the person. Hence impairments are necessary (but not sufficient) conditions for a person to have a disability.

The definition of disability and handicap given by Nordenfelt is this:

> A disability, as well as a handicap, is a non-ability – given a specified set of circumstances – to realize one or more of one's vital goals (or any of its necessary conditions) (Nordenfelt, 1993a, p.22).

Let us focus just on disability for the moment. As seen, disabilities fall within the class of non-abilities; specifically those which derive from factors intrinsic to the person. (So too do handicaps; as with disabilities, those handicaps which are the 'consequences of disease' will be accompanied by impairments.)

The relevance of circumstances seems plain. There's a clear relationship between circumstances and disabilities. To see this, reflect briefly upon the way in which possession of abilities presupposes some contextual factors. For example, if the force of gravity increases I may not be able to raise my arm. Or if one's arm is tied down, one may not be able to move it. More trivially, if there are no books one cannot read. Attribution of a disability to a person similarly presupposes some reference to circumstances. If, at a particular time, a person with paraplegia is unable to stand it is presupposed that the attempt occurs in circumstances in which a non-disabled person could stand if they tried – there is not a gale force wind blowing that is strong enough to prevent anyone from standing etc. And if it is judged that a person has a disability such that they are unable to move their fingers, this presupposes circumstances in which their fingers are not bound together to prevent them from moving.

As seen, the definition also invokes the idea of a 'vital goal'. By this, Nordenfelt means 'a state of affairs that is a necessary condition for the realization of A's at least minimal happiness' (Nordenfelt, 1993a, p.20). It is made plain that vital goals may include activities which are important to an individual such as birdwatching. They also include more physiologically based needs necessary for survival (such as needs for oxygen and water), since satisfaction of these is clearly a necessary condition for the realisation of the goal of birdwatching and so on.

So a person has a disability in a specific set of circumstances if they are, due to the disability, unable to pursue their vital goals.

The category of disabilities is further articulated in terms of what Nordenfelt calls 'basic actions'. Basic actions are 'simple intentional movements of one's limbs or other parts of one's body' (Nordenfelt, 1993, p.22). Thus an action such as making a cup of tea would be composed of the performance of several basic actions. If one is, due to intrinsic factors, unable to perform the basic actions necessary for tea-making, and if tea-making is one of one's 'vital goals', and there are no exceptional circumstances (no hurricane-force winds blowing), then one has a disability.

Nordenfelt thus proposes that a disability is a non-ability to perform a basic action. As he puts it:

> A is disabled with respect to action H, if and only if H is a basic action. A is unable to perform H, given a specified set of circumstances that have been agreed upon in the context. A's performance of H is a necessary condition for the realization of one or more of A's vital goals (Nordenfelt, 1993a, p.23).

So, suppose it is necessary to grasp a cup in order to make tea and that the grasping constitutes a basic action, 'action H'. If circumstances are standard, and not exceptional, and if performance of H is necessary for the realisation of one of a person's vital goals, then that person is disabled with respect to basic actions of the kind just described – that is, grasping actions.

With regard to the class of handicaps, Nordenfelt defines these also, as we saw, in terms of non-abilities to realise vital goals, or the necessary conditions of their realisation. Whereas disabilities are defined in terms of a person's non-ability to perform basic actions, handicaps are defined in terms of a person's non-ability to perform what he terms generated actions. Crudely, the difference between these is that generated actions such as making tea are typically achieved by performance of a chain of basic actions. In the tea-making example, such basic actions would include, as we saw, picking up the necessary implements, and placing them in the appropriate position.

> A is handicapped with respect to action H, if and only if: H is a generated action. A is unable to perform H, given a specified set of circumstances that have been agreed upon in the context. A's performance of H is a necessary condition for the realisation of one or more of A's vital goals (Nordenfelt, 1993a, p.23).

Thus if A is 'unable to board a bus', and being able to board a bus is necessary for A to realise her vital goals, then A is handicapped in circumstances C. The reference to 'circumstances which have been agreed upon in the context' is worth a brief comment here. To stick with the 'boarding a bus' example, suppose the society in which A lives is one in which women are not permitted to travel on buses. It could then be claimed that A is handicapped with respect to the action 'boarding a bus' if this is crucial to attainment of her vital goals. However, this kind of 'social handicap' (Nordenfelt, 1993a, p.20) differs from the kind of handicaps which are our main concern, namely those which are related in some intimate way to factors intrinsic to the person (as Nordenfelt puts it: 'handicaps that are attributable to internal processes' (Nordenfelt, 1993a, p.20)).[5]

Nordenfelt and the ICIDH

As seen in our discussion of the ICIDH the relevant 'goal terms' specified there include, in the case of disabilities, the performance of activities 'within the range considered normal for a human being' (WHO 1980/1993, ICIDH, p.28). And in the case of handicaps the goal terms specified there include 'the fulfilment of a role that is normal (depending on age, sex, and social and cultural factors) for that indi-

---

[5]A key feature of Nordenfelt's approach is its exploitation of action theory. The concept of ability, is subjected to a three-fold analysis. Thus actions manifested in abilities involve an actor, a goal and a set of circumstances. An act of making tea involves the actor, the goal of making tea, and the circumstances in which the tea is being made. Naturally, circumstances may hinder the achievement of the goal, e.g. if there is no electricity or gas supply etc. So Nordenfelt suggests the following analysis of ability: 'When A is able to reach G in C, then [A] reaches G in C if [A] tries' (Nordenfelt, 1993, p.18). So A has the ability to achieve the goal of making tea in circumstances C when A both wants to do so and does so. The analysis of *ability* invites a similarly three-fold analysis of *disability*. In this 'when A is unable to reach G in C, then A does not reach G in C if A tries' (ibid.).

vidual' (WHO 1980/1993, ICIDH, p.29). By 'goal terms' here I mean the kinds of actions – goals of individuals – considered central to the question of whether or not they have a disability or a handicap.

The term 'normal' as it figures in these definitions of disability and handicap is either one of statistical normality or relates to behavioural norms deriving from views about how people ought to act. So the ICIDH approach to defining disability and handicap ties the definitions of disability and handicap to activities or roles which are statistically normal or considered positively desirable in the relevant cultural context.

By contrast, the significance of Nordenfelt's approach is that the goal term is tailored to the vital goals of particular individuals as opposed to general norms (whether statistical, descriptive or normative). Thus its very considerable importance is that definitions of disability and handicap are not separated from individuals' own views about what is important to them in their own lives.

Hence Nordenfelt's approach poses the question of why we should link incidence of disability to what people normally do (in the statistical sense of 'normally') as the ICIDH does, and proposes instead that we should define disability and handicap in relation to an individual's self-chosen goals. A person is then disabled or handicapped if, and only if, they are unable to obtain such goals (and they have an impairment).

To give an example of how this might work out in practice, recall Nordenfelt's example of birdwatching. Suppose this is a vital goal of someone, and further that that person is unable to walk due to paraplegia. That person would be classified as having both a disability and a handicap according to the ICIDH criteria, for walking is an activity 'within the range considered normal...' etc and lack of the ability to walk would be considered to generate a handicap. But according to Nordenfelt's theory, such a person might not be categorised as disabled or handicapped. If they are able to meet all their vital goals and the necessary conditions for achievement of these, in their circumstances, the person would be neither disabled nor handicapped. So Nordenfelt's approach seems not to ride roughshod over individuals' own views about what is important to them in the way in which the ICIDH view does.

Also, recall the criticism raised by the UPIAS that medical analyses of disablement fail to pay sufficient attention to the views of people with disabilities. Nordenfelt's approach is plainly immune from such a criticism since the question of whether or not a person is disabled or handicapped can only be answered by reference to the person concerned, providing they are able to express a view. To my mind, this constitutes a major attraction of Nordenfelt's approach to disablement in comparison with that presented in the ICIDH.

Before closing discussion of it, it is important to clarify further the role of circumstances in Nordenfelt's account. Consider two nation states. One is extremely rich and can boast of a system of social support for its citizens which far exceeds standards available in any contemporary society. The other is much less wealthy and provides only minimal levels of social support. Consider now a person in the rich country who has a serious intellectual disability. The rich country provides the person with a comfortable place to live and 24-hour personal support available every day. Such levels of support are available to all disabled persons in that country. Hence 'standard circumstances' in this society are ones in which such levels of support are the norm.

Providing the person in this state is able to meet all their vital goals, such a person is not disabled (or handicapped) according to Nordenfelt's theory. For 'accepted circumstances' (Nordenfelt, 1995, p.212) here are such that they include the availability of 24-hour support.[6]

Consider the same person in the less rich country. Here there is no 24-hour support and the person is not able to meet their vital goals. Suppose one of the person's vital goals is to visit the cinema every day. In the rich country the availability of constant support makes it possible for the person to do just that. But in the poorer country the lack of support – 'accepted circumstances' – makes visits to the cinema a rarity. Thus the person is not able to meet one of her vital goals and thus renders her handicapped. Obviously, here the handicap stems from the combination of internal factors (intellectual impairment) and external factors (presence/absence of social support).

These examples illustrate once again the role circumstances can play in definitions of disablement, and pointedly they show that political decisions in the form of decisions about social policy have a

---

[6]Nordenfelt defines accepted circumstances thus: 'By "accepted" I mean that the circumstances are accepted by the person who ascribes ability or disability to another person. These circumstances may be standard in the sense of being commonly accepted in a particular culture but they need not be' (Nordenfelt, 1996, pp.180–1).

direct relationship to the incidence of disability and handicap, in Nordenfelt's definition at least. For many people will have the capacity to attain their vital goals given relevant social support. But if this support is lacking, due to lack of political will, they will remain disabled.

Problems with the theory

There are a couple of potential problems with the theory, which Nordenfelt anticipates and tries to deal with. (Recall that his theory of disability is part of a more general theory of health.)

The first of these concerns a person who has vital goals which are apparently at odds with their health, for example a drug addict. On one reading it looks as though Nordenfelt's theory allows that such a person is healthy providing they are able to meet the vital goal of obtaining addictive drugs. Nordenfelt denies his theory has such an implication. His claim is that vital goals are not simply identical with a person's desires or wants (Nordenfelt, 1993a, p.20; 1999, p.183). They are defined in terms of conditions which are necessary for the person's 'minimal happiness in the long run' (Nordenfelt, 1993a, p.20). The implication is that the drug addict's desires are contrary to his vital goals, since fulfilling the desires won't contribute to his long-term happiness.

We might think that is an open question, especially if the drug addict finds it easy to obtain the drugs he wants. But Nordenfelt's approach is such that attainment of vital goals is sufficient for at least minimal happiness since they are defined in terms of minimal happiness. So the attempt to find a problem case for Nordenfelt's theory, in which pursuit of vital goals conflicts with attainment of happiness, simply cannot succeed. This is a matter of logic, given his definition of vital goals.

The second possible problem stems from the way in which disablement is 'individualised' in Nordenfelt's theory. As mentioned, this is part of its appeal. But individualisation may come at a price. Scientific and policy analyses of disablement require the possibility of generalisations. Does not Nordenfelt's approach fatally compromise such analyses?

His response is to point to wide *de facto* convergence in vital goals, concerning pursuit of things necessary for life (water, food, shelter and so on). Ultimately, though, of course, questions regarding the incidence of disability and handicap cannot be 'read off' from a person's physical constitution or appearance.

A third problem, which Nordenfelt does not anticipate as far as I am aware, is as follows. We have seen the definition of disability that Nordenfelt presents. According to it, one is not disabled if one is able to meet one's vital goals. But consider a situation in which a person is able to perform, say, a basic action such as grasping a cup but can do so only very slowly. Suppose this person is, nonetheless able to meet their vital goals. Nordenfelt's view is again in tension with the ICIDH in relation to such a case. For such a person would be disabled on the ICIDH view, but is not on Nordenfelt's. Against Nordenfelt, it seems plausible to say of such a person that they are indeed disadvantaged when it comes to pursuance of their vital goals. Tasks which take others moments take them much longer. (It may be that Nordenfelt's references to 'specified circumstances' can help here.)

There is also the difficulty raised by people who have unrealistic vital goals. Suppose a 95-year-old man claims to be handicapped because he cannot run 100 metres in under 10 seconds. In defence of Nordenfelt, one can point out that such a vital goal is not a reasonable one in those circumstances, assuming, that is, that the man lives in a contemporary western society, and not some future society in which it is common, due to genetic enhancement, for 95 year olds to run at such speeds. Also, of course, there is no impairment present in the 95 year old, so he cannot fall within the class of people with a disability (at least on the grounds claimed).

Finally, it should be added that in English-speaking countries the term 'handicap' is not considered appropriate to use, for reasons of political sensitivity. But this is not, obviously, a serious objection to Nordenfelt's theory. He could simply amend it, using a term less politically charged than 'handicap' (*see* Edwards, 1998; Nordenfelt, 1999 on this specific issue). I will follow the WHO and continue to use 'disablement' as an umbrella term covering both disability and handicap.

Overall, for reasons just discussed, Nordenfelt's theory seems the most adequate considered thus far, and we will return to discuss it following discussion of our last two theories, the first of which is a briefly stated position presented by Professor John Harris.

Harris' definition of disability

Professor John Harris (1998, 2000) has also offered a definition of disability. He defines disability as a 'harmed condition', a condition 'we have a strong rational preference not to be in' (Harris, 2000, p.97).

In a discussion of deafness Harris proposes that the harm this brings is 'the deprivation of worthwhile experience' (Harris, 2000, p.98). A dimension of experience is available to hearing people that is not available to deaf people. (It may be said in response to this that being deaf similarly is a dimension of human experience not available to hearing people.)

The idea that disability deprives people of an important dimension of human experience works least problematically in relation to sensory disabilities such as deafness. But how does it apply to people with moderate intellectual disability and no accompanying sensory disabilities? I suppose it may be said that a moderately intellectually disabled person misses out on those dimensions of experience that require considerable intellectual acumen: these might include doing complex work in physics, maths or philosophy. But of course it could be said of those of average intelligence that they too miss out on such experiences. And it may be said of those without musical ability that they miss out on that dimension of human experience, and so on. The point is, it does not follow from the fact that if one is constitutionally incapable of experiencing certain possible aspects of human experience that one is in a harmed condition.

So Harris' definition is objectionable on at least two counts. First, it is over-inclusive (includes people who are not credibly regarded as disabled). It is so in the sense that it includes people who are not musically gifted, and who lack a very subtle palate. Both such groups of people are 'deprived' of the experiences of playing complex music, or appreciating subtle tastes. As seen, such people are disabled on Harris' line because they are deprived of worthwhile experiences and therefore in a harmed condition. However, neither are credibly regarded as disabled, not least because there is no impairment present.

According to Harris' definition, anyone who, due to 'constitutional factors' (matters of one's physical constitution) is unable to undergo certain kinds of worthwhile experience, such as play beautiful, complex music or solve complex mathematical problems, is disabled.

In fact, since no human is completely able (can do everything) it follows from Harris' definition that all human beings are disabled.

If one thinks of disabled people as a politically identifiable group in the 'disability rights' sense, this is certainly false. Also, if it is true that disablement is a relative concept, and is defined by reference to a contrast class, then Harris' definition empties the concept of any content, for acceptance of it would entail there is no 'contrast class', since all humans would fall within the class of disabled individuals.

A second criticism is that his definition is overly inclusive in another way. The last criticism concerned the way in which Harris' definition includes many groups of people not currently regarded as disabled. Indeed, as we saw, it includes all human beings. But what of people who have disabilities according, say, to the ICIDH definition, but who lead full and happy lives? On Harris' criteria such people are disabled. This is in spite of the fact that, as mentioned, they may be leading full and happy lives. Moreover, it is possible they might, as a consequence of their disability, develop greater sensitivity to certain kinds of experience, perhaps musical experiences they are unable to see. Thus those people defined as disabled when this is conventionally understood (by the ICIDH definition) may not consider themselves disabled, and may be able in dimensions of experience not typically recognised (as in the 'greater sensitivity' example).

Harris' definition, and the criticisms just discussed, lead to a fundamental point in discussion of disability. This is the question of who is best placed to determine whether or not a person is in fact in a 'harmed condition'. Suppose (controversially to some) it is accepted that disability is a harmed condition. Might not a person defined as disabled according to ICIDH criteria, and by Harris, deny they are in a harmed state? If so how should this denial be responded to?

By Harris/ICIDH criteria there is no question of the person's response being accepted: such a person is simply mistaken. But is harm something which can be determined in such a way? It could be argued that the question of whether or not a person is in a harmed condition is at least partly answerable to that person's view of the matter. This is not to say that the person's view will always be decisive. But it must surely carry some considerable weight in any credible answer to the question.

This point lends further support to Nordenfelt's position. In that, as we saw, if a person can meet all their vital goals, they cannot credibly be considered disabled. Similarly Nordenfelt's line allows that such a person could not credibly be considered to be in a harmed condition (if they can meet all their vital goals).

Lastly, strictly speaking, it could not be said that Harris does in fact provide a definition of disability. He identifies only one aspect of such a definition, a necessary condition of any such definition. Thus any definition of disability must categorise it as a harmed condition. But not all harmed conditions are disabilities. Loss of a finger nail might cause momentary pain, and thus amount to a harm. But such a loss does not amount to a disability. Hence Harris identifies at best a necessary condition of disability, but no sufficient conditions. An adequate definition should provide both.

So Harris' position seems open to several serious objections, not least that at best it is seriously incomplete. It identifies only a necessary condition of disability and even that is so contentious as to be very implausible. Let us now turn to discuss the last theory to be considered here, once more provided by the WHO.

The World Health Organization's revised definition of disablement: the *International Classification of Functioning, Disability and Health* (ICF) (World Health Organization, 2001)

In response to some of the criticisms which the ICIDH document attracted, the WHO produced a new classificatory schema for the phenomenon of disablement. In some respects the new schema is similar to the original ICIDH one, and in others it differs from it.

A key respect in which the new document is similar to the ICIDH lies in its definitions of three of its main categories. The prior three-fold classification of impairment, disability and handicap is replaced with impairment, activity limitations, and participation restrictions. So previously we would have impairment (e.g. an abnormality in anatomical structure such as a missing spinal nerve), leading to disability (inability to walk), and to handicap (e.g. inability to work). Now we have impairments, activity limitations, and participation restrictions. These are still taken to concern body parts and functions, the person, and the social context respectively (WHO, 2001, p.188).

Impairment is defined as follows:

> Impairment is a loss or abnormality in body structure or physiological function (including mental functions). Abnormality here is used strictly to refer to a significant variation from established statistical norms (i.e. as a deviation from a standard population mean...) (WHO, 2001, p.190).

It is evident that this definition is not substantially different from that which appears in the ICIDH. The focus is on body parts, functions, and statistical abnormalities in structure or function. As mentioned in our discussion of the ICIDH, such aspects of the person are the focus of biomedical models of disease.

To try to clarify the relationship between disease and impairment, it is said that impairments differ from 'underlying pathology' (diseases) but are, rather the 'manifestations' of that pathology (WHO, 2001, p.16). So a degenerating optic nerve would be an example of 'underlying pathology' and the impairment it would generate would be difficulty in seeing. Here, then, the disease generates the impairment. But it is also pointed out that impairments may be present, even though a disease is not (WHO, 2001, p.17), the example given here is of a person who loses a leg, an injury as it might be put. Such a person has an impairment but not necessarily a disease (say, if the loss occurred as a consequence of an accident as opposed to a circulatory disease).

So, given acceptance of the claim that loss of a leg through injury is not a disease, we can see that impairments are related only contingently to diseases. The latter may generate impairments, but impairments may be present in the absence of disease. As will be seen, though, an impairment is a necessary condition for the presence of a disability – though not a sufficient condition (a person may be impaired but not disabled). Nor does the presence of an impairment necessarily indicate ill-health.

Some impairments are not associated with disabilities. Myopia need not be a disability, given availability of appropriate 'facilitators' such as spectacles.

The disability dimension of the ICIDH, the 'person level' dimension, is defined thus:

> Activity limitations are difficulties an individual may have in executing activities. An activity limitation may range from a slight to a severe deviation in terms of quality or quantity in

executing the activity in a manner or to the extent that is expected of people without the health condition (WHO, 2001, p.191).

Note that the explicit reference to 'activities within the range considered normal for a human being' is now deleted. But of course it is still there implicitly in the reference to 'people without the health condition', though this can now be considered more specifically in terms of people within the social context of the person as opposed to human beings *per se* (as is indicated in this quote: 'Limitations or restrictions are assessed against a generally accepted population standard' (WHO, 2001, p.21)). Note too that reduction in the quality of performance of an activity is mentioned within the definition. So if one can still grasp a cup but can do so much more slowly than one used to, and much more slowly than other people, one counts as having an activity limitation.

The more 'social' dimension of disablement is represented by the term 'participation restriction', and this is defined thus:

Participation restrictions are problems an individual may experience in involvement in life situations. The presence of a participation restriction is determined by comparing an individual's participation to that which is expected of an individual without disability in that culture or society (WHO, 2001, p.191).

So, as with the ICIDH category 'handicap', it appears that a participation restriction is determined by reference to the typical kinds of activities engaged in by one's peers. If one is restricted from engaging in such activities, due to impairments or activity limitations, one suffers from a participation restriction.

At each of the three levels, differing responses may be appropriate. At the level of impairments, medical responses may be called for. At the level of activity limitations, physiotherapy or provision of therapeutic aids may be appropriate (use of a stick in a blind person, or a speaking device for communication as used by Stephen Hawking). And at the level of participation restrictions, changes to the social environment may be the appropriate response. This may take the form of introduction of 'facilitators'. These are 'factors in a person's environment that, through their absence or presence, improve functioning and reduce disability...' (WHO, 2001, p.192).

The authors of the ICF are at pains to stress that disablement is not conceived of solely as a problem of the individual. The role of environmental factors is made plain: hence, 'a person's functioning and disability is conceived as a dynamic interaction between health conditions (diseases, disorders...) and contextual factors' (WHO, 2001, p.10). To signal this, it is made explicit that the ICF involves a rejection of a medical model of disability, without embracing a social model. Instead a model which recognises a role for both kinds of factors is adopted. As they put it 'a "biopsychosocial" approach is used' (p.28). In other words, one which takes into account factors at the three levels of analysis identified earlier and formerly captured, however obscurely, by impairment, disability and handicap.

It is also stressed that the 'consequences of disease' approach has been jettisoned too (WHO, 2001, p.5). Instead a 'components of health' schema is adopted which 'takes a neutral stand with regard to aetiology...' (WHO, 2001, p.5). Thus, it does not presuppose that, for example, impairments make one less healthy.

To take an example: consider a person with visual difficulties. According to the ICF, 'body functions are the physiological functions of body systems (including psychological function)' (WHO, 2001, p.15). Thus digestion would be a body function, as would respiration and cognition. And 'body functions include basic human senses such as "seeing functions" and their structural correlates exist in the form of "eye and related structures"' (WHO, 2001, p.15). So a person with visual difficulties may have a disorder of body function if their optic nerve is not functioning properly, and this stems from a disorder of body structure.

'Body structures are anatomical parts of the body such as organs, limbs and their components' (WHO, 2001, p.15). Thus a limb counts as a body structure. An eye would count as a body structure (though p.15 is hard to interpret on this specific point) '...impairments are not the same as the underlying pathology, but are manifestations of that pathology' (WHO, 2001, p.16). 'Impairments are problems in body function or structure as a significant deviation or loss' (WHO, 2001, p.111). So an impairment would thus stem from a relevant bodily structure (such as a missing or damaged part of the eye or surrounding structures such as the optic nerve).

Hence we could conclude that visual difficulties would satisfy the definition of an impairment. The impairment may be linked to an 'activity limitation', e.g. the activity of 'watching' or other 'purposeful sensing' (WHO, 2001, p.123). And in turn it may be linked to a 'participation restriction' such as watching TV or, more seriously, a reduction in the range of career opportunities open to the person (e.g. medicine).

With regard to intellectual disabilities, a person may have an impairment (loss or abnormality of psychological function). This may be associated with an activity limitation (problem solving or some other function of cognition 'learning and applying knowledge' (WHO, 2001, p.19)). And this in turn may be associated with a participation restriction (in that certain activities typical in one's peer social group may not be open to one, such as playing chess, or pursuing study at an advanced level).

As we saw, the ICF notes that participation restrictions can be alleviated by devices, such as powered wheelchairs, or changes to the social environment, such as changes to public transport to make them more wheelchair friendly (WHO, 2001, p.20): so-called facilitators.

Summary of the main differences between the ICF and the earlier ICIDH

- The ICF 'provides a multi-perspective approach to the classification of functioning and disability as an interactive and evolutionary process' (WHO, 2001, p.25). It takes into account the person themselves, their body and their views, together with their physical and social environments. It 'is based on an integration of [the medical and social] models. In order to capture the integration of the various perspectives of functioning, a "biopsychosocial" approach is used' (WHO, 2001, p.28). This, by implication, concedes that the ICIDH placed insufficient emphasis on external factors, and on 'non-medical' factors generally.
- Impairment is not now the fundamental category in the ICF (Bickenbach *et al.*, 1999, p.16). Again, by implication, this suggests that impairment *was* the 'fundamental category' in the ICIDH, though, as indicated in our discussion of the ICIDH above, this may stem from an unsympathetic reading of it.
- 'Disability' now has very broad usage: 'Disability is an umbrella

term for impairments, activity limitations and participation restrictions. It denotes the negative aspects of the interaction between an individual (with a health condition) and that individual's contextual factors (environmental and personal factors)' (WHO, 2001, p.190, *see also* p.3)

The analysis presented in the ICF is broad in another way also. It is said to embrace a 'principle of universality' and to reject a 'minority group' analysis of disablement (*see* Bickenbach *et al.*, 1999). What is being claimed is that 'Disablement ... is an intrinsic feature of the human condition, not a difference that essentially marks one subpopulation off from another' (Bickenbach *et al.*, 1999, p.17).

Thus rather than convey a view in which disabled people form a discrete and easily identifiable minority group, the 'principle of universalism' points up the universality of the experience of disability. No human being is able in every respect, and disablement is experienced by a great many, perhaps all, human beings. There are two further points about the ICF that deserve comment; these relate to universalism and the clash between the WHO definitions and Nordenfelt's theory.

The universalism of the ICF

For most humans, disablement is temporary in the form of illness and so on. It is true that our powers decline in older age, but it is not clear that this decline is accurately regarded as disabling. If it is the case that disabilities require impairments, and if impairments are defined in terms of 'species typicality' (and are relative to age and social context), then it is not clear that such decline legitimately counts as disability.

(Note too how the assumption of universalism bears upon screening programmes designed to reduce the incidence of disabling conditions. If disability is a universal trait, and if screening programmes aim to reduce disabling traits, we are not far from the conclusion that no births should be permitted to occur!)

The assumption of universalism is a striking introduction in the light of the way in which, as a political strategy, disability rights campaigners have tried to articulate a distinct 'disability identity' (UPIAS, 1975). This was observed earlier in relation to some remarks made by Oliver (1990) and other commentators. In the works of such commentators, disability is promoted as being politically on a par with sex and race. Hence to discriminate against disabled people because of their disability is morally equivalent to discriminating against people on grounds of their sex or ethnic origin. But the adoption of the principle of universalism plainly subverts that political tactic. For according to this principle all humans are disabled, or will be at some stage in their lives. This would be like responding to racism by stating that all humans belong to the same race, or to sexism by claiming all humans are of the same sex.

We will be discussing the relationship between disability and identity in a later chapter so we will not pursue that now. But one point can be aired. Is it legitimate to claim equivalence between 'ableism', sexism and racism? In support of such an equivalence claim, the relationship between disability and income and other social factors such as unemployment may be pointed to. It may be claimed that just as legislation was needed to outlaw discrimination on grounds of sex or ethnicity, so too legislation was needed to outlaw discrimination against disabled people (again, *see* UPIAS, 1975).

In consideration of such a claim it is important to acknowledge at the outset that discrimination is unjust. In fact it is best understood as a violation of a principle of justice according to which 'equals should be treated equally and unequals should be treated unequally' (Aristotle: Beauchamp and Childress, 2001, p.227). To give an example, suppose a lecturer gives all the male students in his class top marks, but no female student obtains top marks. When asked to explain, the lecturer says he never gives female students top marks, even when, of course, a female student's work merits such a mark. Here is a clear case in which the principle of justice is being violated. Equals are not being treated equally in the sense that not all students who produce high-quality work are awarded the same grade. The justification offered for this is plainly inadequate. He focuses on an aspect of the situation which is not morally relevant, this being the sex of the student. All that should be considered morally relevant is the quality of the student's work (not the sex of its author). The lecturer's role is to assess the quality of the work submitted and award it the appropriate grade. The sex of the person who presented the work is plainly irrelevant. To put this more technically, the sex of the student *is not* a morally relevant characteristic in this situation. The quality of the work done *is* morally relevant.

Legislation aimed at ruling out discrimination is intended to prohibit judgements which distinguish against people in ways that violate the principle of justice. Hence it need not rule out *all* decisions that involve judging between people, only those that stem from considerations that are not morally relevant, and thereby unjust.

To give an example, in the UK people with severe visual impairments are not currently able to become physicians. They are not permitted to train as doctors and so are barred from medical practice. Suppose two equally qualified students apply to medical school. One of the students has a severe visual impairment and the other has no discernible disabilities. The medical school decides to accept the latter student and not the former. The decision, it may be claimed, involves no contravention of the principle of justice because it is made on the basis of a characteristic credibly deemed to be morally relevant in this case, this being the difference in visual capacity of the two applicants.

Thus it can be seen that decisions that distinguish between persons *need not* involve violations of the principle of justice. They may be defensible by appeal to that principle. Of course, there is room to debate the question of whether severe visual impairment *should* be considered a morally relevant characteristic in this context. It may be argued that medical schools should be prepared to take students with such impairments. But that is a debate which need not concern us here. It is being supposed here, for the sake of argument, that the UK policy is defensible. Consideration of its application in the example just discussed shows that judgements which involve distinctions between individuals (or even groups of individuals) need not involve violations of the principle of justice.

So in situations in which having a disability *is* a morally relevant characteristic – as, perhaps, in the example just given – it may be morally defensible to distinguish between people on grounds of disability. But in situations in which having a disability is not a morally relevant characteristic, then judgements which exclude disabled people *do* constitute violations of the principle of justice.

Hence 'ableism' is a coherent concept, and indeed morally on a par with sexism, racism and ageism. However, it does not follow from this that we should regard disability as conceptually equivalent to race and sex. The reason is that disability, in contrast to race and sex, is always accompanied by impairment. To say this is not necessarily to say that disability is a 'consequence of disease'. Rather, it is to say that impairment is a necessary condition of disability. And further, the proposal that impairment is a necessary condition of disability falls short of claiming that it is a sufficient condition: a person may have an impairment but not be disabled (or even ill).

Plainly, neither being female nor being a member of an ethnic minority can be regarded as an impairment. But disability can be shown to be related to the presence of impairment within an individual. This may be genetic, or structural (as in the 'optic nerve' example), or physiological (e.g. relating to abnormal metabolism).

Bickenbach et al. (1999) make the point that it is indeed important to show why certain characteristics are associated with social disadvantages and injustice. In order to distinguish disadvantage due to disability from disadvantage due to sex or race, it is necessary to point to the role which impairment has in the phenomenon of disablement. As they put it:

> The nature of the link between impairment and disablement is an important issue for any social theory of disablement, since without some researchable connection it would not be possible to distinguish the socially-created disadvantages of disablement from those of race, gender, class or economic status (Bickenbach et al., 1999, p.6).

So, as argued above, it is a mistake to see 'ableism' as conceptually on the same footing as sexism, ageism, and racism. For ableism stems not from the fact of a person's sex, age or race but from their having a disability. And this will be accompanied by an impairment. Thus there is a key difference between disablement, sex and race. The latter two need not be accompanied by impairment; the former always is.

As just explained, to say this is not to show the concept of 'ableism' is spurious. On the contrary, our discussion above showed how judgements can be ableist in violating the principle of justice by improperly regarding disablement as a morally relevant property. (Recall too that disablement can sometimes be morally relevant, as the 'medical school' example above shows.)

The point of identifying the strong connection between impairment and disablement is to show that there is a difference between injustices due to racial or sex discrimination, and injustice involving ableism.

The clash between the WHO definitions and Nordenfelt's theory: evaluation

Our discussion of justice, recall, stemmed from our two comments on the ICF. The second point of note concerns the obvious conflict between Nordenfelt's definition of disablement and that put forward in the ICF.

As we saw in discussion of Nordenfelt's view, the question of whether or not a person is disabled or handicapped is bound very closely to that person's own view of the matter. And in the main, the question of whether or not a person has a disability or handicap depends upon what is important to that particular person. It is tempting to describe Nordenfelt's approach as a subjectivist one because of the emphasis placed upon the views of the person whose disability is in question. But he has rebutted such charges convincingly (Nordenfelt, 1999). According to his theory, although the views of the person concerned count for a great deal, they are constrained by some independent considerations, relating to that person's longer-term happiness and quality of life. So let us accept that Nordenfelt provides an adequate basic account of disablement. In this, as we saw, x is disabled if x cannot realise relevant vital goals in standard, specified circumstances.

If we compare this to the WHO's two definitions there is a clear conflict. A conflict arises with the ICIDH definition since, as seen, this binds definitions of handicap to statistical norms concerning role fulfilment. And the ICF definition of participation restrictions (i.e. disabilities) defines these by reference to roles 'expected of an individual without disability in that culture or society' (WHO, 2001, p.191).

For Nordenfelt, disability is defined by reference to individual goals. Statistical norms are irrelevant – at the levels of disability and handicap at least (though perhaps not at the level of impairments since these hinge upon definitions of disease which may rest upon statistical norms relating to biological structure and function). Thus it can be seen that Nordenfelt's definition is at odds with both WHO definitions. They rest upon statistical norms, his rests upon an individual's view of what their vital goals are.

To give a concrete illustration of the difference between the two approaches, consider the UK Member of Parliament (and former

Home Secretary) David Blunkett. He has a severe visual impairment. By Nordenfelt's definition, if Blunkett can attain his vital goals he is neither disabled nor handicapped. But by either of the WHO definitions Blunkett is categorised as either handicapped or disabled. By the ICIDH definition he is handicapped since blindness disrupts a person's capacity to fulfil a statistically normal social role. And by the ICF, as the medical school example given above shows, blindness generates a 'participation restriction' at least as far as entry into that profession is concerned.

Is there any way of adjudicating between the two approaches? It is agreed by the WHO and by Nordenfelt that disablement is significant due to its relationship to health status. Nordenfelt's theory of health is very similar to his theory of disability. So, for him, health also is defined broadly in terms of ability to meet vital goals. In this way it can be seen to have at least two very significant aspects. The first is its evaluative nature. As with disability, health is inseparable from the capacity of an individual to seek and fulfil states which are important to them, or to put the same point slightly differently, to attain states which the individual *values* (hence the claim that this is an evaluative theory of health). The WHO also, famously, propounded a theory of health which includes a key value-laden concept, that of wellbeing. ('Health is a state of complete physical, mental and social well-being and not merely the absence of disease or infirmity' (WHO, 1946).)

So it is fair to say that both definitions, those of the WHO and of Nordenfelt, are evaluative in nature, indeed Nordenfelt explicitly describes his theory as such. So the difference between the two parties – WHO and Nordenfelt – is not one of philosophical substance at this level: both regard health as an evaluative concept.

The difference lies in the extent to which what is a health matter, in the broadest of senses, should be a matter of mainly individual concern, or mainly determined by statistical norms. As seen, Nordenfelt's line is that this is mainly an individual matter. The choice of particular vital goals is, by and large, personal. If a person has an unusual choice of vital goal, the non-ability to pursue it could still count as a disability or handicap.[7]

---

[7]As we saw, though, there are some constraints on what can count as a vital goal for Nordenfelt: it must connect up with a person's 'long-term happiness', and is constrained by 'standard circumstances' so it cannot be unduly extravagant or unduly meagre (Nordenfelt, 1999).

It will be argued here that there are in fact good reasons to favour Nordenfelt's approach over that of the WHO. A philosophical case for this will be mounted when we look (in Part Three) at the relationship between disability and the person. But part of the case can be signalled here. Recent years have seen a growth in the recognition of the importance of personal narrative in the context of healthcare (Kleinman, 1988; Greenhalgh and Hurwitz, 1998). This is central to diagnostic and preventative work in the following way.

A great many health problems are lifestyle related, they include hypertension, heart disease, stomach ulcers and so on. And other conditions have 'lifestyle' elements to them, for example conditions such as asthma and diabetes. Of course an individual's lifestyle is an exemplification of their narrative. Crudely, their behaviour mirrors their pursuit of things they value, whether this is high status via their work, or a secure family life, or a life with many kinds of physical pleasures or a combination of these things, etc. If a disorder of their body – a bodily change which generates a health problem – interrupts a person's capacity to pursue what is important to them, then that physical change disrupts the person's narrative. Put in Nordenfelt's terms, the disorder jeopardises their pursuit of their vital goals. Thus it is that illnesses have a 'personal' element to them. These points strongly suggest the importance of personal narrative in diagnosis of health problems.

With reference to preventative work, of course it may well be that a personal narrative makes it more rather than less likely that a person will become ill. Hence preventative medicine will require close understanding of patients' values and goals, in other words, their narratives.

If these claims concerning the importance of individuals' narratives are accepted, they lend support to Nordenfelt's position as it applies to disablement. They do so because health and illness are ultimately bound up with pursuit of goals which are part of a patient's narrative. Since there is no reason to assume all people will share the same narrative, the categories of health and illness must be sensitive to individual variation. Nordenfelt's definitions of both health and disability do this, as we saw above. The WHO definitions, by contrast, are ultimately grounded in statistical norms. This, in my view, lends greater weight to Nordenfelt's theory of disablement over that proposed by the WHO.

Responses to (anticipated) criticism

Some comments on the preceding conclusion are needed now. Many theorists of disablement will be disappointed about the analysis just presented. It reinforces the view of disablement as a state within the general medical sphere. It does so because it sees disablement as a health-related state, necessarily associated with an impairment.

It is being supposed here that properties of individual persons which we normally classify as diseases are typically disvalued. There may be exceptions (Sedgwick's example of spiro chromatosis (1982)), but in the main they are properties human beings would prefer not to instance. Considerations such as these generate the claim that disease states are indeed value laden: they are states we generally disvalue. This of course leads us straight into a controversy, because many people with disabilities detect a chain of reasoning here which they find offensive and harmful to their interests. Roughly, the chain runs as follows:

> If disabilities are always related in some way to the presence of impairments; and if these in turn stem from diseases (or other states, such as injuries); and if diseases (and other such states which qualify as impairments) are disvalued states; then people with disabilities are disvalued.

In addition, attempts to define disability which are conceptually linked with definitions of health reinforce two objectionable impressions. First that disability is a medical concern – that the 'medicalisation' of disability, and the medical model of it are appropriate. And second, that disability is always accompanied by ill-health.

All three of these objections require serious consideration and response:

- that defining disabilities by reference to disvalued states implies that people with disabilities are disvalued
- that regarding impairments as necessary conditions of disability unduly medicalises disability
- that regarding impairments as necessary conditions of disability entails the claim that disabling conditions inevitably compromise a person's health.

Before dealing with these three points, some further clarification is required concerning disease and impairment. Regarding disease. As noted, minimally, diseases are disvalued states. It then follows that those impairments that are generated by diseases are too. Also, the kinds of conditions which are impairments but not diseases – call them maladies – such as injuries, are plausibly regarded as disvalued states. That is why we seek to prevent the occurrence of maladies such as amputated limbs, that is the point of health and safety at work legislation and safety features in cars and other forms of transportation.

What else can be said about such disvalued states? They cannot adequately be defined by reference to statistical norms. Some abnormal states are neither diseases nor disvalued, e.g. having red hair. Moreover, some statistically normal states may well be both disvalued and diseases, e.g. tooth decay, and obesity in some parts of the world. For a state to count as a disease, or as a malady, some at least potentially adverse functional effect is necessary. Such effects on function may be at the level of the person conceived of as a biological organism. It does not follow from this that diseases will adversely affect the capacity of the person considered to function as a person – as more than a biological organism.

So two necessary conditions of diseases, and also of impairments will be posited here. The first is that any such state is a state which is typically disvalued. The second is that any such state is a state which adversely affects the function of the individual considered as a biological organism.

It is important to note the intentional use of the phrase 'biological organism' here. This is to leave room for discussion of function at two levels, so to speak. The first is the biological level. The second is what we can term the narrative level. This latter level concerns the person's values, intentions, goals, relationships and so on. The purpose of the distinction is to allow the possibility of disruption of function at the biological level, which does not impact adversely upon function at the narrative level.

To give an example, consider again David Blunkett. Here it can be said that at the biological level, there is an absence of function of key elements of a key sensing system, the visual system. So at this level there is an impairment, which results in the absence of a key function. This can be said without it implying that, at the narrative level, Blunkett has a disability. That question remains to be answered.

Also, RF Murphy, in his description of life with a progressive degenerative disease of the nervous system, states that in the early stages of the condition he didn't regard himself as disabled because he remained able to do those things which mattered most to him (Murphy, 1987, p.70). In other words, he could fulfil his vital goals.

With this clarification completed, let us return to the three concerns raised above.

The objection to conceptually locating disablement in the health sphere mentioned above, is that this implies that people with disabilities are themselves disvalued. I will spend more time dealing with this objection later, since its acceptance trades upon the view that disabilities can be 'identity constituting' (Part Three). But an initial response to it is called for now. The response is this. The fact that a disabling condition is disvalued *need not* entail that the person with that disability is disvalued. A person with multiple sclerosis (MS) may disvalue that condition (*see* Toombs, 1995), and it may be disvalued by others – as exemplified by the quest for a cure for MS – but that person may still be valued. So the mere location of disability within the conceptual sphere of health need not entail that people with disabilities are disvalued.

Moreover, suppose it could be shown that people with disabilities are, as a matter of empirical fact, disvalued, in the sense that they are the victims of social exclusion. From a philosophical perspective, the pertinent question is whether or not this exclusion is defensible. If it is not, a position emerges which recognises that people with disabilities are disvalued, but provides resources for a case to show this is morally objectionable – for example on the grounds that such disvaluing is the result of a violation of the principle of justice.

So this first objection has met with two responses. The fact that disabling conditions are disvalued need not entail that people with those conditions are disvalued. And second, if people are disvalued due to their disability, this is not sufficient for the moral defensibility of such practices; indeed, such a practice would count as 'ableism'.

What of the second objection. The criticism here is that of the medicalisation of disablement. What does the charge of medicalisation amount to? As we heard above in discussion of the ICIDH it involves these claims: (a) the causes of disability lie within the individual; (b) the locus of attention in amelioration of disability should be the individual; (c) the identification of disabling traits is a medical matter (especially when the question of the presence or absence of such traits is linked to accessibility to social benefits etc). With regard to (a), it is now clear that this is false. The most probable proposal is that the causes of disablement are at least two-fold, partly due to the social environment, and partly due to the presence within an individual of an impairment. The response just offered to (a) addresses the concern raised in (b) also. For if the causes of disability do not reside solely in the individual, then the locus of attention should not exclusively be placed upon the individual. The nature of the social environment needs to be considered too (as stated in the ICF). Finally, in response to (c), in part this is a matter of social convention. Matters relating to the bodies of people – as impairments are properties of bodies – are, as a matter of social convention, the terrain of medical personnel, or their close cousins such as dentists and optometrists. And given that impairments either are, or stem from, diseases and injuries, it seems unavoidable that some medical involvement will be required to diagnose the presence of an impairment. Even if not medical, then something closely related to the medical sphere will be relevant here, as in dentistry, or optometry.

It should be stressed that defending the case for medical involvement (even in the broader sense just identified) in diagnosis of impairment does not entail a similar role for detection of disability. Given the social component of disablement, and its intimate relationship to the narrative/values of the person concerned, a role for other persons is needed here.

The third suggestion is that locating disablement in the sphere of health equates disability with ill-health. But this charge too can be resisted. In response, consider the distinction between illness and disease. A virus, for example, is an instance of a disease, a disease-entity as we might say. A person may have a disease-entity within their bodily system, but feel fine. It can be said of such a person that they have the disease but do not feel ill. Suppose the person begins to feel the effects of the viral infection, she feels tired, hot and struggles to get through her daily routine. Now, according to this distinction, the person feels ill. Thus disease is defined in terms of anomalies of function, lesions, or in terms of disease entities such as viruses. But illness is defined in terms of how a person feels.

If we apply this distinction to the context of disability, it is plain that a person may have an impairment but not feel ill – think of the David Blunkett example given previously, or that of Jenny Morris. But having said this, some disabling conditions may well, at least for long periods, cause the sufferer to feel ill. MS may be a useful example of such a condition, as may Lesch–Nyhan syndrome. So while it is important not to equate disabling conditions with illness, one should be careful not to overstate the case and to fail to recognise that some disabling conditions do cause long periods of ill-health. Hence, although the relationship between disability and illness is indeed a contingent one, strictly speaking, some disabling conditions are closely connected with feelings of illness, indeed they cause them (as in MS).

Conclusion

As seen, then, Nordenfelt's general theory of disablement has been considered here in relation to its main rivals. And in spite of the kinds of likely objections to it as considered in the last section, it has been endorsed here. But there is a dimension of the analysis of disablement which, in my opinion, Nordenfelt's theory neglects. This is the distinction between capacities and abilities which was explained on p.13.

Thus Nordenfelt's theory of disablement can be supplemented as follows. A disability with respect to action A is still a non-ability due to some impairment within the person. Some of those non-abilities will stem from loss of the capacity to perform A, and some will stem from non-ability where the person retains the capacity to perform A.

The distinction is important. For in cases where a person's (P) non-ability to perform A stems from an impairment, one can pose the question 'Does P have the capacity to perform A?'. If the person does have the capacity to perform A but not (at present) the ability to perform A, then the possibility of interventions to facilitate P's development of the ability to perform A is opened up (e.g. by 'facilitators' or physiotherapy or education, etc). Of course, if the person does not have the capacity to perform A (say if A is a 'basic action' in Norden-felt's sense), different interventions may be indicated.

In this chapter, then, we began by considering just why it seems important to have definition of disablement. And following considera-tion of rival definitions, Nordenfelt's theory was found to be the most defensible. Towards the close of the chapter, the theory was defended from anticipated objections (regarding the medicalisation of disable-ment etc) and was supplemented with the ability/capacity distinction. It is worth stressing again that Nordenfelt's theory is very sensitive to individual life plans. So, strictly speaking, the presence of an impairment in an individual (including foetuses) is not sufficient for their having a handicap (in Nordenfelt's sense) or for their being disabled. So the contingency between the presence of an impairment in an individual, and the question of their disablement, is given a further layer by acceptance of Nordenfelt's theory.

A first layer of contingency obtains in that a person may have an impairment but not a disability (as we saw the UPIAS, ICIDH and ICF also endorse this). A second layer of contingency between impairment and disability is presented by the social context. As we heard, for proponents of the social model, certain changes in the social context can 'evaporate' certain disabilities. So this presents a second layer of contingency between impairment and disablement. The third layer is brought about by Nordenfelt's theory which shows the presence of an impairment may not be disabling if it does not impugn a person's pursuit of their vital goals. And this is something they are best placed to determine.

Given all this, how should prenatal screening programmes be thought of? The question is especially cogent given the close relationship between such programmes and rates of termination. Adoption of Nordenfelt's theory shows how the presence of an impairment in a foetus may not generate a disabling trait. It should be stressed that this is a point made in the ICIDH, the ICF, and by the UPIAS too. Moreover, the reason why an impairment generates a disabling trait may be more connected to the social environment than to the impairment – as emphasised in the social model.

These layers of contingency – as I have termed them – prompt consideration of the grounds for termination of pregnancy when a genetic impairment associated with disabling traits is detected in the foetus. Thus the topic of Part Two concerns prenatal screening and the conception of a good human life.

PART TWO

Disablement and the idea of a good human life

Introduction

Discussion of the nature of disablement showed that impairments are not sufficient conditions of disabilities. The question of whether or not a person has a disability cannot be 'read off' from their physical characteristics. As in Nordenfelt's theory of disablement the person's own view of the matter is relevant to the question of whether or not they have a disability (Nordenfelt, 1993a). The presence of genetic (or structural) anomalies can be diagnosed prenatally. But acceptance of Nordenfelt's definition of disablement shows that disablement cannot be determined prenatally. So, while the presence of impairments can be detected prenatally – in the form of genetic or structural anomalies – disablement cannot be. For the question of whether an impairment generates disablement will be dependent upon that person's own view, in conjunction with other external contingencies (such as the nature of the person's social environment). Very strictly speaking, then, the issue of prenatal screening and diagnosis, with consequent terminations of pregnancy on grounds of disabling traits in the foetus should be recast as one involving prenatal screening and diagnosis of *impairments* (and not disabilities). Having made this point, for ease of exposition, I will continue to speak of termination on grounds of disability in the foetus, for that is what people engaging in such a practice take themselves to be doing.

The point of addressing the relationship between disablement and the idea of a good human life is this. As will be shown, decisions to terminate a pregnancy when prenatal diagnosis reveals a genetic anomaly associated with a condition interpreted as disabling (e.g. Down's syndrome), are taken against a background of presuppositions regarding what counts as a good human life.

51

We saw in Part One that in the UK and elsewhere the practice of prenatal screening and diagnosis is generally acknowledged to be a good one, and that it is closely allied to rates of termination when disabling traits are detected.

Before showing how such decisions presuppose a conception of a good human life, two comments are worth making on the practice of prenatal genetic diagnosis (PGD).

First, disabilities can be physical, intellectual, or sensory, and within these broad categories there are extremely wide ranges in degree of severity of a disability. For example, Down's syndrome can cause very severe intellectual disability with many accompanying physical problems, or very mild intellectual disability with relatively few physical problems.

The severity of the disability cannot be read off from the genetic information. This is the case with Down's syndrome, and also with neural tube anomalies, amongst other conditions such as fragile X.

Second, as we have seen, the definition of disability is itself contested. It is possible to identify at least five different definitions of disability (Union of the Physically Impaired Against Segregation (UPIAS), 1975; World Health Organization (WHO), 1980, 2001; Nordenfelt, 1993a; and Harris, 2000).

These two considerations suggest that great caution should be exercised before decisions to expand screening programmes are made. Because, although the programmes aim at genetically diagnosable impairments, due to the three-fold contingent nature of the relationship between impairment and disablement, the presence of an impairment need not entail that the person has a disability.

What we will do in this part of the discussion, then, is first to try to show that decisions to terminate pregnancy are made against tacit presuppositions concerning what counts as a good human life. This will be illustrated making use of a 'real life' case in which a person describes the reasons for terminating a pregnancy upon learning that the foetus has Down's syndrome. We will then look at three main philosophical theories of what counts as a good human life and look at the decision to terminate from the perspective of each of the theories. The discussion will show that most disabilities are compatible with the conditions necessary for leading a good human life. And, more contentiously, it will be argued that disabling conditions need not inhibit a person's capacity to lead a good life.

Termination of pregnancy and the idea of a good life

It is plausible to claim that what lies behind decisions to terminate a pregnancy when allegedly disabling traits are diagnosed is a conception of what constitutes a *good human life*. Parents standardly have some idea – if only implicitly – about what kind of a life they would like their children to lead. A decision to terminate on grounds of an impairment in the foetus betrays some view of what counts as a good life.

To see this, I will 'invent' a horrific genetically based syndrome. It bears some similarity to Lesch–Nyhan syndrome, but is designed to entail a life even worse than life with that. I will call the hypothetical syndrome, Syndrome Z. Furthermore, I will constantly refer back to this hypothetical syndrome throughout the rest of the book. Here it is:

> Syndrome Z: a diagnosable genetic anomaly is known to cause syndrome Z. Life with this syndrome is short (maximum of 10 years), is accompanied by very serious intellectual disability, and constant, unremitting, unrelievable pain. This is thought to explain the self-injurious behaviour which always accompanies syndrome Z.

Why might a prospective parent decide not to proceed with a pregnancy in which syndrome Z is detected? In the specific case of syndrome Z, a description of the symptoms of the condition would very likely be accepted as an adequate answer to the question.

But suppose it is asked further 'Why is a life with those symptoms considered so bad?'. It is at this stage that tacit assumptions regarding what is and what is not compatible with leading a good human life begin to become explicit. For it would surely be responded that it is not possible to lead a good human life – under any credible conception of what such a life might be – while enduring the symptoms of syndrome Z.

It looks as if life with syndrome Z is incompatible with the conditions necessary for leading a good human life. A person with syndrome Z lacks the very *capacity* to lead a good human life, is *constitutionally incapable* of leading such a life, and is so due entirely to *intrinsic factors*.

It is true of course that life with syndrome Z is still life, and, therefore, in the eyes of some, of great value. But even if this is accepted, it does not follow that life with syndrome Z is a *good* life. Indeed, one may think it morally abhorrent to claim that it could be. For such a life involves futile suffering, suffering without any counterbalancing features.

It should be stressed again that this is a hypothetical syndrome, to be used here for purposes of exposition. However, the case for the claim that decisions to terminate pregnancy when disabling traits are diagnosed in the foetus presuppose conceptions of a good human life will be supported also by the following actual case (*see also* Baily, 2000).

A woman named Emma Loach described in a newspaper article why she decided to terminate her pregnancy upon learning that her 20-week-old foetus had Down's syndrome (*The Guardian*, 5 June, 2003). She received medical advice from her consultant physician to the effect that, due to the presence of Down's syndrome, her child would have a short life expectancy (30–40 years), would have constant medical problems, and would never be independent. Also, she was told a Down's syndrome child would impose a severe burden upon the lives of herself and her partner, and upon their existing child. She describes how, upon hearing these predictions, she decided, together with her partner, to terminate the pregnancy.

The inaccuracy of these claims about life with Down's syndrome, for present purposes, can be set aside. What is important is their moral relevance as perceived by Emma Loach. It is her child's prospects as she understands them, rather than as they actually are that motivate her decision to terminate the pregnancy. The key considerations as she relates them, in the order in which she relates them, run thus:

> Life expectancy of 30 or 40. Never being able to look after himself. Likely to have serious medical problems all his life. Also [her existing son] Samuel ... would have a completely different childhood with such an ill sibling. And Elliot [Loach's partner] and I would have a completely different life from the one we'd imagined (Loach, 2003, p.2).

Let us now consider these grounds more slowly, focusing first on the factors that concern the prospective child. The relatively low life expectancy is considered significant. The clear implication is that longer life expectancy is considered preferable. But why is this?

One plausible reason is that a longer life expectancy, one closer to the average length of life (say, in the UK since Emma Loach's decision was taken there), gives a person longer to complete a 'self-project' (*see also*, Part Three for development of this idea). Such a project may include career aspirations, having a family, leisure pursuits and so on. A life-span closer to the average provides more time to complete this. A shorter one runs a greater risk of leaving the project incomplete.

In support of the claim that these considerations expose implicit presuppositions concerning what counts as a good human life, the presupposition here is that a longer life provides greater opportunity to lead a good life. A life which is 'cut short' so to speak is 'less good', in a sense to be made clear, than one which continues to the normal life span or beyond.

These ideas are not unproblematic of course. A person aged 80 may feel they have not yet completed a 'self-project', and never will since it is constantly being developed and revised, and a younger person may well feel their own life project has been completed during their 40s, say. Nonetheless, in Emma Loach's case, the clear implication seems to be that a low life expectancy is disvalued. If asked why, it seems reasonable to suppose that the kinds of considerations rehearsed in the previous paragraph would emerge as significant.

Turning now to the second element of the medical advice which appears in the quote, pertaining to the prospective child. Here the absence of independence is feared ('Never being able to look after himself'). This is thought to be so even with respect to the most basic of daily activities. No further details are provided in the passage, or even in the article as a whole on this specific point. But 'never being able to look after himself' covers, potentially, a very wide range of meanings. At one extreme, it may mean he will not be capable of the most basic personal hygiene, such as washing, dressing and eating. Or, that he may be able to do these things but be incapable of living without supervision, independently. Whichever point along this broad spectrum Loach envisages, it is fair to summarise her fear in terms of *independence*. The child will always lack independence, and will therefore be dependent upon others even when an adult.

As with the role played by life-span in Loach's decision, the tacit appeals to independence and dependence can be queried. Strictly speaking, humans simply are interdependent, typically. In an obvious sense they are dependent upon other human beings for their very existence, and nurturing in early years. And even when they are adults, they seek the company and stimulus of other humans. So, strictly speaking of course all humans are dependent upon others, and even well into adulthood they remain so, typically.

One suspects that Loach would agree with these points but, perfectly reasonably, would object that they don't do justice to her line of reasoning. She could legitimately point to a sense of 'dependence' compatible with these suggestions about the origin and social nature of humans and still maintain that a severely intellectually disabled adult would be *excessively* dependent. They would be dependent in the usual ways, but have a further dimension or layer of dependence due to their disability. This further 'layer' would entail that they could not be economically independent – relative to their peers – in a way in which intellectually able people do have the ability to be.

The role which the concepts of dependence and independence have in conceptions of disablement will be taken up in more detail later (Part Three). But it is interesting that they lie close to the surface in Emma Loach's reasoning. The clear implication is that a life which involves excessive *dependence* upon others, even loved ones, is not as good a life as one in which a person has greater capacity for independence, specifically, when this is understood in economic terms.

The third claim made by Emma's consultant, again with reference to the prospective child, is that a life with Down's syndrome is 'likely' to be accompanied by lifelong 'serious medical problems'. Once more, these are not specified in the article, but it is reasonable to suppose Emma would associate such a proposal with the need for very frequent medical attention, requiring many hospital admissions and procedures.

Still focusing solely on the prospective child, it is reasonable to assume the constant need for medical attention will be associated with considerable suffering on the part of the child. Such suffering will stem from the inherent pain and discomfort of undergoing surgical procedures, the stress of hospital admissions and the fear evoked by the anticipation of such admissions. In other words, the consultant is telling Emma Loach her child will suffer throughout his life, not least from the sources just identified.

Place these points in the context of the claim that Emma's decision presupposes a conception of a good human life. It is perfectly reasonable for Emma to infer, from the medical information she is provided with, that the prospective child's life will be filled with suffering, of an awful kind, a kind associated with interminable, serious health problems. And it is reasonable for us to infer that this again indicates a conception of what counts as a good human life. A good life, it is implied, does not involve the kinds of excesses of suffering which will befall her prospective child – again, as she infers from the medical advice.

Taken together, then, it is being proposed here that these considerations contribute significantly to Emma Loach's decision to terminate her pregnancy. As presented within the article it is not clear whether any of the three considerations is considered weightier than the others, or whether it is the fact of all three that led her to opt for termination. For our purposes, the significant factor is that each of the considerations impacts upon the prospective child's capacity to pursue a good human life, at least as far as Emma Loach is concerned.

Let us unpack the quoted passage still further. Whereas the first three considerations focus on the prospective child, the fourth brings in the effects on Emma's existing child, Samuel. The phrase runs he 'would have a completely different childhood with such an ill sibling'. Strictly speaking, this may be interpreted in at least two ways. First one could suggest that Samuel's childhood, though *different*, will be better than it would otherwise have been. However, it is very unlikely, given the tenor of the rest of the quote and the eventual decision, that the statement is interpreted like this. More likely, the statement is intended to signal adverse consequences for Samuel. For example, that he will have less of his parents' attention than he would otherwise have had, for they will be preoccupied with his sibling and his 'constant medical problems'. Also, Samuel will miss out on the fun of having a non-disabled brother, and may suffer social stigma and teasing from his peers due to his having a brother with Down's syndrome.

These suggestions also connect up with ideas of what is a good human life. The clear message is that if the pregnancy is to proceed Samuel's life will not be as good as it could have been. The presence of a sibling with Down's syndrome is considered to inhibit Samuel's chances of leading a good life (however this is conceived of).

The final consideration referred to in the quote concerns the parents, Emma and her partner Elliot. Again the exact phrase ('Elliot and I would have a completely different life from the one we'd imagined') is, strictly speaking, neutral in its predictions about the effects of a Down's syndrome child upon their lifestyles. The phrase *could* be read positively or negatively. But as with the part referring to Samuel, the context of the quote as a whole, plus the decision to end the pregnancy can be taken to indicate that the birth of the child is expected to bring negative, not positive effects.

Once again, it is plausible to relate these grounds for termination with the idea of a good human life. This time, the lives concerned are those of the prospective parents. Having to deal with a severely disabled, constantly ill child will inhibit their capacity to pursue a good life, by their lights.[1]

This time spent unpacking Emma Loach's grounds for termination, briefly stated as they are in the original article, is with the goal of supporting the claim that such decisions stem from background presuppositions concerning what counts as a good life. The preceding discussion succeeds in doing this, in my view, and it shows that the considerations rehearsed show concern for the capacity of the prospective child, his sibling, Samuel, and of course his parents Emma and Elliott to lead a good life.

It is reasonable to conclude, then, that decisions to terminate pregnancy on grounds of a disabling trait within the foetus presuppose some conception of a good human life. Emma Loach's conception is such that a good life doesn't involve continual suffering and dependence.

If it is indeed true as argued here that decisions to terminate when disabling traits are diagnosed rest upon conceptions of a good life, it will be important to consider carefully what is meant by the expression 'good human life'. For if there are different conceptions of this, then we might reach differing judgements about whether or not life with a particular impairment is incompatible with, or impedes the prospects of leading such a life. Also, if it is true that conceptions of a good human life inform judgements about termination of pregnancy where disablement is detected in the foetus, surely it will be important to spell out such conceptions further. This will help ensure that deci-

---

[1]For research to support the view that having a disabled child as a family member disrupts parents' lifestyles adversely, see the report of the Canadian government survey in the *Toronto Star* (30 July 2003, bioethics@egroups.com, 31 July 2003). For other views, see Ferguson *et al.* (2000) and Reinders (2000).

sions to terminate on such grounds really are autonomous in the sense of being adequately informed by relevant considerations.

It should be stressed that 'good' in this context need not (though it may) mean a life full of 'doing good', a good life in the sense in which one might say of a saint that they led a good life – a life comprising countless good deeds. There is another perfectly familiar – if rather vague – idea of a good life. This is appealed to when one says of another 'they led a good life', or of one's children 'I hope they have a good life'. In this other idea, a good life may be thought to include at least some of the following: pleasure, fulfilment, family life and friendship.

In order to try to pin down a bit more precisely just what a good life might involve, it may be useful to turn to some philosophical work on that very question. A survey of such work (Aristotle, *Nichomachean Ethics*; Griffin, 1986; Parfit, 1986, pp.493–502; Elster and Roemer, 1991; Brock, 1993; Nussbaum and Sen, 1993) reveals that there are three main theories, each of which attempts to answer the question 'What makes a good human life?'.

The theories are helpfully labelled as follows by Brock (1993): (a) hedonistic; (b) preference satisfaction; and (c) ideal (for reasons that will become evident, I'll call ideal theories 'objective goods' theories).

A hedonistic theory of the good life

Although I will speak of one theory, strictly speaking there are a cluster of theories coming under this title. But what they each have in common is a focus on the subjective experience of the person.[2]

On this approach to the question, a good human life is one consisting of a great many pleasurable experiences. These might include experiences such as sexual pleasure, the pleasure of achieving a treasured goal (attaining a doctorate, or passing a driving test, or scoring a cup-winning goal for England and so on), or gustatory pleasures.

It is vital to note that this theory focuses on the mere *experience* involved in the kinds pleasures just described. The reason this is

---

[2]Such theories are associated with the Greek philosopher, Epicurus 341–270 BC. Crudely, as an approach to ethics, hedonism maintains that pleasure is the good. So acts which maximise pleasure are morally justified. A good life is one which involves attainment of pleasure. More recently, it is associated with the utilitarianism of the 18th century philosopher Jeremy Bentham (1748–1832).

significant is because, clearly, one might have the experience of having achieved x without actually having achieved it. So the focus of this theory is not on actual achievement, only on subjective mental experiences. On this view, one's life is improved by undergoing pleasurable experiences and made worse by being deprived of them.

Consider now how the hedonistic conception might apply in the context of disablement. Many conditions thought to be disabling are not incompatible with the undergoing of pleasurable experiences. Down's syndrome would be one of several possible examples. Only conditions such as the hypothetical syndrome Z would plainly be incompatible with the conditions necessary for leading a good life as this is considered within a hedonistic approach.

By the lights of this theory, then, disablement need not prohibit one from meeting the conditions necessary for leading a good life, in principle. Syndrome Z of course does entail that, in principle, it is not possible for one to lead a good life.

It is important, before moving on, to be clear about what is being claimed when advancing this kind of judgement. As noted, it is possible for a person to have Down's syndrome and to lead a good human life as this is understood within a hedonistic theory. But in saying post-mortem that a person lived a good life by hedonistic standards, what, strictly speaking, is claimed? I take it that it would be being claimed that the person had a sufficient quantity of pleasurable experiences to merit that judgement. This must be more than just one pleasurable experience one would suppose. A life with just one pleasurable experience couldn't count as a good human life by the hedonistic criterion. Strictly speaking, the theory only allows us to conclude that such a life would have been better if a greater quantity of pleasurable experiences had been undergone.

If it is true that a life with no pleasurable experiences won't count as a good life by a hedonistic theory, and that a life with just one, sole, pleasurable experience isn't either, we seem forced to posit a certain quantity of pleasurable experiences the undergoing of which will be sufficient for attainment of a good human life. In other words we seem forced to assume a *threshold* of pleasurable experiences, attainment of which entails that one led a good life, and failure to attain which entails that one did not.

But surely specifying such a threshold is an impossible task. For suppose it is said that a life with N pleasurable experiences is a good life. It seems perfectly reasonable to ask why a life in which N minus

1 experiences are undergone could not also count as a good life. If one concedes that such a life should indeed count as a good life, then one faces the same problem. If a life with N minus 1 experiences can count as a good life, why not a life with N minus 2, and so on, and so on ... This regress appears to have no principled stopping point. It might be said that a life with only one pleasurable experience is still better than no life at all. But this point is not really one directed to the question of what is a good life. Its proper target is the question of whether it is better to live than not to live, when only one pleasurable mental event is experienced. This question is separable from ours, which is 'what is a good human life within hedonistic theory?'.

Assuming, then that a good life within a hedonistic theory requires experiencing at least two pleasurable experiences – we are forced to allow this due to the difficulties involved in specifying a threshold – it can be allowed that life with very many conditions currently regarded as disabling can be a good life. In addition, this discussion shows the difficulty in attempting to specify any kind of threshold quantity of pleasurable experiences sufficient for leading a good life. Any posited quantity can always be queried and is then vulnerable to regress.

This difficulty is a little puzzling since, presumably, when one judges a life, post-mortem so to speak, one is typically doing so against a presumed threshold (within the hedonistic approach at any rate). So at the theoretical level, the idea of a threshold is extremely problematic. Yet, in practice, retrospective judgements about the goodness of a life, from the hedonistic perspective, must invoke one.

In focusing on pleasurable experiences, we have omitted to mention painful or otherwise unpleasant experiences. Judging the goodness of a life within hedonistic theory surely requires consideration of these. For suppose a person has N pleasurable experiences and N plus 1 painful ones, a net loss in terms of pleasure overall. Is this a good life? I think we would have to conclude such a life could not be a good life in the terms of hedonistic theory, for there a good life is a pleasurable one. If a life involves more pain than pleasure it cannot be described as a pleasurable life, overall – *even though it may have involved the experience of pleasures.*

A further consideration is that of length of life. This may be thought relevant to the present discussion since some disabling conditions are associated with a shorter life span, for example Down's syndrome and cystic fibrosis. But this should not be relevant from the hedonistic perspective. What matters is one's capacity to endure pleasurable experiences, and the quantity of these that one experiences. A longer life need not entail a life with more pleasurable experiences. For, suppose it is true that a person with Down's syndrome typically dies between the ages of 50 and 60 whereas a person without Down's syndrome typically lives over 10 years longer. The person without Down's syndrome has more years to accumulate more pleasurable experiences it may be said.

However, of course the extra life years experienced by the person without Down's syndrome give that person more years to accumulate *unpleasant* experiences too. So we can't straightforwardly assume that more life years equals more pleasure and therefore a better life. Also the person with Down's syndrome may well have experienced extremely high levels of pleasurable experiences but only a few displeasurable experiences prior to his death.

Lastly there are well-known difficulties with the general problems involved in the comparison and quantification of pleasure and pain. For example, how can one compare the pleasure of listening to a Beethoven late quartet with that of seeing one's football team win the FA Cup? Is it feasible to suppose these could be analysed within the same frame of reference and then quantified? I think in general, this has not been taken to be a feasible task. And even if one could accomplish this within a single person, it seems doubtful that one could accurately do so across persons and develop an inter-personal scale so to speak (Nordenfelt, 1993b, pp.23–32).

These points are all intended to make clearer what is involved in a judgement of the form 'x had a good life' when this is made by the standards of hedonistic theory.

By way of further clarification, some enquiry needs to be made as to the sources of pleasure that a person experiences. To take Down's syndrome again, there is no incompatibility between life with this and the experience of pleasure.

Also, it is reasonable to propose that a significant range of sources of pleasure are prompted by events external to the person. These might include gustatory pleasures after being presented with tasty food, those stemming from achievement of a goal, those resulting from involvement in relationships, and so on. In typical cases, a significant range of pleasurable experiences have an external cause. Certainly, the list of examples of types of pleasures just given are such causes. Of course, some pleasures need not have external causes, mental and sexual self-stimulation being two such kinds.

Suppose now we ask the question: 'will x have a good life?', in the knowledge that x has an impairment associated with some kind of disabling condition, and that we are considering the question within the framework of hedonistic theory.

We can set aside conditions such as syndrome Z for there is no prospect of leading a good life with this condition, when a good life is understood as it is in a hedonistic theory. The above discussion shows that the question of whether x will lead a good human life depends to a significant degree upon external contingencies. It is certain that a person with Down's syndrome has at least the capacity to lead a good life, since that condition does not preclude pleasurable experiences. These range from the kinds of love and support x can expect from family members, and social structures. Now surely this is the case for any child whatsoever (at least those without syndrome Z, or any equivalently awful or worse condition).

It was shown above that decisions to terminate pregnancy on grounds of disabling traits within the foetus presuppose judgements about what counts as a good life. From the perspective of hedonistic theory, it is not the case that having a disabling trait is incompatible with leading a good life (excepting syndrome Z and any cognate conditions). And the question of how likely a child is to lead a good human life depends upon external contingencies. This seems morally on a par with what is the case for healthy foetuses. They have the capacity to lead a good human life. Whether or not they will do so depends upon what happens outside the womb. Does this entail, then, that decisions such as that taken by Emma Loach above are made on mistaken grounds?

Well, if her decision stemmed solely from consideration of the prospective life of the Down's syndrome child, it looks as if it is mistaken (*when viewed from the perspective of hedonistic theory*), for the prospects for leading a good human life, as conceived of within hedonistic theory, are no different from the prospects of a non-disabled child. This conclusion is warranted due to problems with the quantification of pleasurable experiences, and the contingency between greater life expectancy and the having of an increased amount of pleasurable experiences.

Recall, however, that Emma Loach's decision also takes into account the effects on her existing child, Samuel and upon herself and her partner. Consider Samuel first. Our question is, 'could Samuel lead a good human life, by the lights of hedonistic theory, if he has a younger brother with Down's syndrome?'. The clear answer to this is that there is no necessary incompatibility between Samuel's capacity to lead a good life while having a brother with Down's syndrome. For obvious reasons, it remains possible for him to have pleasurable experiences. Of course Samuel may not get on with his brother, but again this is possible whether or not his brother has Down's syndrome. As with the prospective Down's syndrome child, the chances of Samuel leading a good life are determined by external contingencies.

Turning now to Emma Loach and her partner. Again, there is plainly no incompatibility between having a Down's syndrome child and leading a good life, by the lights of hedonistic theory. The question of whether they will or not do so is dependent upon external contingencies, just as it would be if the child did not have Down's syndrome.

The claims just made suggest there is little difference between a decision to have a disabled child (providing the disability is not syndrome Z) – specifically one with Down's syndrome – and to have a child with no disabling traits. There is little difference because in each case (a) there is no incompatibility between capacity to lead a good life and the presence of disability, and (b) whether or not one actually leads a good life hinges upon external contingencies. Both (a) and (b) are true whether one's focus lies on the disabled child, on existing sibling(s), or the parents. These are not trivial claims; their significance should be dwelt upon.

These conclusions are likely to generate two responses. The first is that the 'external contingencies' referred to above can be divided into two spheres, the 'domestic sphere' over which the child's parents will have more control, and the 'public sphere' over which the parents obviously have much less control.

The second response is that the discussion above has been operating with a 'threshold' approach to the issue when a differing approach is called for. This other approach may be called a 'maximising' approach. So, the response runs, although it is true there is no incompatibility between life with disability and the criteria for leading a good human life, the presence of disability obstructs opportunities to lead a maximally good life. We will come back to this later, but for now we return to deal with the first response (that regarding domestic and public spheres).

Public/domestic spheres

Consider, then, the first response. It should be said in advance that the distinction between two domains, public and domestic is a rather rough and ready one. Obviously, the public sphere impacts upon the domestic one. If social conditions are poor, with high rates of poverty and unemployment, plus high mortgage interest rates, it may be much more difficult to provide the 'external contingencies' referred to above. In spite of this, though, there is a clear sense in which the nature of the domestic sphere is amenable to more influence by its members than the public sphere. A family can decide to do more or less together. Parents can decide how much time to spend with their children (again subject to the proviso given above regarding the separation of domestic and public spheres), and how much of the family budget to spend on family entertainment, relationship building etc.

The response may continue thus. It may well be true that the family has the capacity to generate conditions necessary for the leading of a good human life (within hedonistic theory, as we have heard, this is the capacity for undergoing of pleasurable experiences). But these will not be sufficient. When the capacity of all family members is taken into account, it is evident that some resources from the public sphere will be required. Such resources, in the case of Emma Loach for example, may include educational support for her child when he begins school. This may be necessary throughout his school career and even beyond.

If Emma and her partner are sufficiently wealthy, they may be in a position to ensure this support is in place. These requirements can be covered by resources available within the domestic sphere. But, if Emma and her partner Elliot are not able to pay for this support themselves (assuming their child needs it, which he *might not*), their child's capacity for leading a good life is at the mercy of public funding. This boils down to taxation. It takes us into questions of distributive justice and the nature of the state. We will need to return to these questions later in Part Two but we won't pursue them at this stage of the discussion.

Also, of course, within the public sphere it may be that stigmatising attitudes to Down's syndrome would impair the prospective child's capacity to lead a good life.

But what we can conclude from discussion of this first response is this. As shown above, Emma Loach's prospective child has the capacity to lead a good human life (as this is understood within hedonistic theory). The extent to which the child can manifest this capacity is contingent upon the conditions present in two spheres, domestic and public. Let us now discuss the second response referred to above.

Threshold or maximising?

What of the 'maximising' response? This is a response which, again, will be dealt with in more detail when we have considered all three theories of the good life, but it will be instructive to set it out here. The response runs like this. A disabling condition may not be incompatible with fulfilment of the conditions necessary for leading a good human life. In effect this is what the positing of a 'threshold' amounts to – in spite of its problematic theoretical status. But, the response continues, disability inhibits a person's capacity to lead a maximally good life. In other words, this response allows that a person with a disability may in fact lead a good life. Nonetheless, it is suggested, their life could have been even better were they not disabled (Singer, 1993; Harris, 2000).

In the context of a hedonistic view of a good life, this cashes out as follows. Suppose it had transpired that Emma Loach's foetus had been diagnosed as having an untreatable genetic anomaly which causes deafness. From the maximising perspective, if Emma had continued with the pregnancy and given birth to a deaf child, the child may well have lived a good human life. It may have had sufficient quantities of pleasurable experiences to meet the threshold of such experiences considered sufficient to have led a good life. However, the proponent of the maximising view suggests that the child's deafness inhibits his capacity to lead a maximally good life, to experience yet more pleasurable experiences, most obviously, those that depend upon possession of the sense of hearing. The child won't hear music, the sound of the sea, or the voices of his family. If he could hear, he could experience these pleasures. Therefore, the deafness impairs his capacity to lead a maximally good life, where this means having the capacity to experience as many pleasures as possible (as seen in Part One, this is a line of argument developed by Harris (2000)).

To counter this proposal (that from proponents of a 'maximising approach'), it may be conceded that being deaf does indeed close off one avenue of possible pleasures (those requiring the capacity to hear). But, it may be said, other avenues of possible pleasures are made available, for example, the membership of a thriving deaf community with its own culture and language (*see* e.g. Rée, 1999).

I am not sure how persuasive a response such as this would be to a 'maximiser'. But it does merit consideration. If all that is relevant within hedonistic theory is the experience of pleasures and the capacity to experience them, it is not clear why certain kinds of pleasures should count for more than others. Why should the pleasures obtained from hearing weigh more than those obtained from membership of the deaf community? Also, since, within hedonism, all that counts is experiencing pleasures, why should having more 'avenues' for the receipt of pleasure be considered better than having fewer. After all, the main consideration is the experience of pleasure, not the means by which these experiences are delivered.

These seem to me reasonable responses to the maximiser. In the context of hedonistic theory, with specific reference to deafness, it is hard to sustain the claim that maximal opportunities for experiencing pleasure are diminished. For, though one avenue is closed, others are opened up. And all that matters in the hedonistic line is the capacity to experience pleasure, not that these result from certain kinds of sensory inputs rather than others.

The maximising claim seems even harder to defend in relation to Down's syndrome. Reportedly, people with Down's syndrome have a generally happy disposition, relish and enjoy the company of others, and opportunities for having fun. Surely here it could be argued, the capacity to experience pleasure is, thus, maximised by virtue of having Down's syndrome.

Of course, as discussed above, people with Down's syndrome have on average a shorter life span than those without the condition. But, again as seen above, it cannot be assumed that more life years equals more pleasure. More life years generate greater opportunities to experience pleasure but they present opportunities to experience displeasures too.

In summary, then, before passing on to the next theory of the good life, it has been shown that adoption of hedonistic theory demonstrates no incompatibility between a life with disability and the capacity to lead a good life. Whether or not that capacity is realised is dependent upon external contingencies in domestic and public spheres. Adoption of the maximising perspective does not show convincingly that deafness, for example, hampers a person's capacity to lead a maximally good life. When applied to disabling conditions which are associated with shorter than average life expectancy, such as Down's syndrome, the maximising line does not clearly show capacity to lead a maximally good life is hampered by this feature of the disabling condition, for there is a contingent relationship only between increased life years and increased pleasure. Also, any claims for a necessary relationship between length of life and pleasure may not do justice to considerations such as the *intensity* of the pleasure. It may be claimed that a shorter life, with a capacity for experiencing greater intensity of pleasure, actually involves a greater quantity of pleasure than does a longer life with a capacity to experience only standard intensity of pleasure.

We have postponed a couple of key questions for later. The first concerns the resources and support available in the public sphere, and the second concerns the maximising approach itself. Should this be adopted in decisions to terminate a pregnancy when disabling traits are discovered in the foetus? We will examine this question later.

We turn now to the second of our theories of the good life, preference satisfaction theory.

Preference satisfaction as the good life

As was the case in our discussion of hedonistic theory, there are strictly speaking a cluster of theories falling under this title. But I will refer only to preference satisfaction theory. The key idea here is that a good life consists of having as many of one's preferences or desires (desires and preferences can be regarded as equivalent for present purposes) satisfied as possible. Thus if I have a strong desire to obtain a PhD, my life is better if I actually obtain one. My life is worse if this desire is not satisfied.

The theory has its origins in a specific interpretation of Mill's version of utilitarianism. In this, the most morally defensible course of action aims at maximal satisfaction of preferences, as opposed to maximal increases of pleasure. (*See* his book *Utilitarianism* (Mill, 1861/1962, pp.259, 260, 262); also, Parfit, 1986; and Elster and Hyllard, 1986.)

As mentioned, there are various ways in which this theory has been modified (e.g. Goodin, 1986) but I take it that the general proposal is clear, and indeed that it has good intuitive appeal. The suggestion that one's life goes best when one's desires are met sounds very plausible.

Note that this theory differs importantly from the hedonistic theory. In the latter all that matters is undergoing the *experience* of obtaining a PhD (to stick with this example). And as noted earlier one may have the experience of achieving something without *actually* achieving it (e.g. by hallucination, drug-induced state, or some mad scientist tampering with one's neurological states). On the preference satisfaction theory, one's life only goes better if one's preferences are *actually* satisfied. Merely believing that they are, or having the mental experience that they are, is not sufficient.

Disabling conditions such as syndrome Z prevent the formulation of preferences. In this hypothetical case, we can suppose the extent of intellectual disablement to be so great that preferences cannot even be formulated. If all disabling conditions were like this, it would follow that disablement is always incompatible with leading a good human life, as this is understood within preference satisfaction theory.

But of course most disabling conditions are not akin to syndrome Z. They do not prevent the formulation of preferences by the person. And it is reasonable to suppose that some of these may be satisfied. Take a person with Down's syndrome again. Such a person may have a range of preferences concerning events in their life that are satisfied. If a significant range of these preferences is satisfied then surely the person has a good life by the criterion of a good human life set out in the preference satisfaction theory. So in the light of preference satisfaction theory, Emma Loach's prospective child could have led a good life, assuming that he would have been able both to formulate preferences and to satisfy them. Or, to return to consider the possibility that Emma's foetus is born deaf, here too there is a clear range of preferences that the person would be able to satisfy in spite of being deaf.

So, as with the discussion of hedonistic theory above, we can quickly conclude there is no incompatibility between disability and the conditions necessary for leading a good life within preference satisfaction theory (again, excepting severely intellectually disabling conditions such as syndrome Z).

What if it is proposed that disability impairs one's prospects for leading a maximally good life, in other words for satisfying one's preferences? A difficulty with such a proposal is that one's preferences cannot be known in advance of one's birth. Of course those relating to basic needs, being pain-free, warm, well-fed and so on can reliably be predicted. But large classes of other preferences cannot, such as those relating to personal interests and one's own conception of what a good life is.

Against this line of argument, it is sometimes argued (again as we saw above in Harris' account of disablement) that disabilities are incompatible with leading a good human life since in at least some disabilities a whole range of preferences cannot be satisfied. In such disabilities the condition renders a person constitutionally incapable, so to speak, of satisfying a certain kind of preference. This point is most easily made in relation to sensory disabilities, such as deafness. Here there are a range of preferences involving the use of that sense which a person will never be able to satisfy (hearing the sound of a human voice, or music and so on).

But against this, however, we can make two points. First, if the suggestion is that a good human life requires that hearing-related preferences be satisfied, then this sounds more like an 'ideal' or 'objective goods' theory of a good human life. For it appears to be being claimed that certain preferences are intrinsically good. But this cannot be claimed within preference satisfaction theory. One of the virtues of the theory is that it leaves people free to formulate and seek to satisfy their own preferences, and thus pursue their own conception of what is a good life for them.

Second, it could be asked if it is possible for a deaf person to formulate a preference involving hearing. Just as one might say that a person who has never seen has no conception of what it is to see, so one might say that a person who has never heard has no conception of what it is to hear. If so, they will not be capable of formulating preferences which involve the sense of hearing, and so cannot be claimed to be incapable of satisfying such preferences.

Also preference satisfaction theories are subjective in the sense that they don't prescribe what preferences a person should have. As Mill puts it, famously, one should be free to pursue one's own good in one's own way (Mill, 1859, p.138). It is for each individual to decide what is important to them, which preferences they would like satisfaction of in order for their life to go better. So I think the objection made by Harris can be resisted, certainly as it applies to sensory disabilities.

Moving on to intellectual disabilities, in a response analogous to that made to sensory disabilities, the defender of preference satisfaction theory may claim that a range of preferences is unavailable to the person with intellectual disabilities. It may then be argued that the inability to formulate those specific preferences impairs a person's capacity to lead a good life. Such preferences might be those relating to devising solutions to complex intellectual problems or engaging in complex intellectual activities.

However, this argument also can be contested. 'Complexity' is surely a *relative* concept. What some find simple, others find complex. And disabled or not, many of us experience the process of finding a task difficult at first, due to its complexity, but we then find it simpler as we become used to tackling it. It is perfectly reasonable to suggest that a person with intellectual disabilities can experience the intellectual pleasures of solving intellectual problems, even if these are problems that others might not find so complex. In solving them, the person displays the preference to solve them and the satisfaction of solving them.

So the proposal we have been considering is that disabilities impair a person's capacity to lead a good life, as this is understood within preference satisfaction theory. According to the proposal, disabilities are characteristically accompanied by the unavailability of specific general types of preferences. These may include preferences to hear or see x; or preferences to perform activities of a certain kind (such as complex intellectual tasks). The responses to this proposal set out here are that the proposal is actually not one that the defender of preference satisfaction theory can advance, for it appears to regard certain categories of preference as intrinsically good. The defender of preference satisfaction theory cannot legitimately legislate in advance which types of preference a person ought to try and satisfy.

Also, as we saw, intellectual disabilities are compatible with the formulation of preferences to solve complex problems. This is because complexity is a relative concept. Finally, as with the example of the person with a severe auditory impairment discussed in response to hedonistic theory, it can be argued that sensory (and other) disabilities open up a range of opportunities for satisfaction of potential preferences, for example regarding membership of the deaf community. Or, with reference to severe visual impairment, to increased sensitivity and fine discriminations in other senses such as hearing or touch.

Furthermore, other preferences will still be formulated such as those for pleasurable experiences and maintenance of relationships with family and friends. So without specifying that some kinds of preferences are of intrinsic value it is hard to see how a preference satisfaction theorist can argue that moderate intellectual disability, for example, impairs capacity for preference satisfaction.

Our focus so far within discussion of preference satisfaction theory has been on the prospective disabled child and his prospects for a good life as this is envisioned with preference satisfaction theory. But when we were discussing Emma Loach's decision and the grounds for it, it became evident that concerns for her existing child Samuel, her partner, and herself were all considered relevant. It was argued here that, ultimately, the decision rested against a background of presuppositions concerning what is a good human life. So we now need to consider the perspectives of these three parties within the context of preference satisfaction theory and the extent to which their prospects for leading a good life are jeopardised by having a child with Down's syndrome.

Consider Samuel first. A first point to emphasise is that there is plainly no incompatibility between having a sibling with Down's syndrome and both formulating and satisfying preferences. So the birth of the child would not necessarily impede Samuel's capacity to lead a good life.

Are his prospects for preference satisfaction impaired by the sibling? It is plain that the opinion of Emma and her partner is that this is indeed likely to happen. On the reasonable assumption that Samuel's preferences will include those to spend time with his parents, Emma concludes that these preferences are likely to be frustrated to an unreasonable degree. This will, she supposes, be due to the amount of time she will need to spend with his (prospective) Down's syndrome brother, due both to his special needs and his 'constant medical problems'. Also, one may speculate that, due to the social stigma of having a Down's syndrome sibling, Samuel's preferences not to be socially excluded because of this will also be thwarted. And lastly, he may prefer to have an intellectually able sibling.

In response to these points, even if they are true, it may still be the case that Samuel could satisfy sufficient quantities of preferences, throughout his lifetime, to have a good life. This is, of course, if we adopt the admittedly problematic theoretical (though practically inescapable) idea of a 'threshold' quantity of preferences satisfied during that lifetime.

So within preference satisfaction theory, the birth of a Down's syndrome sibling, is not incompatible with Samuel's capacity to lead a good life. It is possible for Samuel to satisfy sufficient preferences to count as having had a good life. Could the life have been better without the Down's syndrome sibling? In other words, are his prospects for leading a maximally good life impeded by the birth of his brother?

It is very difficult, perhaps overwhelmingly so, to answer a question of this kind, especially within the confines of preference satisfaction theory. As discussed above, that is a *subjective* theory of the good life in that it does not (should not) legislate about the kinds of preferences a person should formulate and seek satisfaction of. So, given uncertainty about Samuel's future preferences, it cannot be concluded they will be adversely affected by the birth of a Down's syndrome sibling. It may transpire that Samuel believes the range of preferences open to him is wider than it would have been without such a sibling. He may become interested in Down's syndrome, the social support networks available for people with that condition and their families. And it may be that his relationship with his sibling has a distinctive character such that he finds it maximises rather than minimises opportunities for preference satisfaction.

These last points all provoke empirical questions, with research available to support points on either side, so to speak. Some research suggests that having an intellectually disabled sibling adversely affects the non-disabled sibling, other research contradicts such findings (*see* Ferguson *et al.*, 2000). Such research also presupposes a conception of the good life. In research which purports to show the adverse effects on siblings of having a disabled brother or sister, the term 'adverse' presupposes some conception of a good human life. For it is only against such a background conception that life events can be described as adverse – or even as positive of course. So the discussion here impacts not simply upon decisions to terminate pregnancy when disabling traits are diagnosed. It also has important ramifications for empirical research into the experiences of families with a disabled member(s).

Turn now to consider the lives of Emma Loach and her partner. In a fundamental respect, it could be claimed, their preferences have not been satisfied by the news that their foetus has Down's syndrome. They would prefer a non-disabled child. Their life has become worse, so to speak, with this news.

But it is important to pause for a moment rather than simply to accept their judgement at face value (the judgement that their life has become worse, since an important preference has not been satisfied). The reason for pausing a moment is to recall the earlier point that Down's syndrome is not an *intrinsically* awful condition. Unlike syndrome Z it is not one which is incompatible with leading a good life. Given this, let us speculate for a moment upon what Emma and her partner would really prefer. This appears easy to answer, they would prefer a *healthy* child, certainly one free from impairments and disabling traits.

Recall, now, our discussions of the nature of disablement in Part One. Disability is not incompatible with health. One can be healthy and have a disability (as this would be understood from a lay perspective) or even within the International Classification of Functioning, Disability and Health (ICF) (WHO, 2001). Also, the discussion of disablement concluded with the view that the question of whether or not a person is disabled cannot be answered independently of the opinion of the person concerned (where they are capable of expressing a view), *pace* the theory proposed by Nordenfelt (1993a). So it follows that it cannot be predicted in advance of the birth of Emma's son that he will be disabled. If he can meet his 'vital goals', as we saw, he is not disabled.

Given acceptance of the view that there is no incompatibility between having a Down's syndrome child and satisfying preferences, it follows that both Emma and her partner retain the capacity to lead a good life (as understood within preference satisfaction theory). With regard to the question of whether they could credibly attain a reasonable 'threshold' of preference satisfaction, the quoted passage we analysed above lends some clues to this question. It is evident from it they would prefer their prospective child (a) not to have Down's syndrome; (b) to have at least an average life span; (c) to be capable of independent living; (d) not to be beset with medical problems; (e) not to adversely affect the life of their current child Samuel; and (f) not to adversely affect their own lives.

We have dealt with the first preference; the second probably will not be met; the third may be met as may the fourth, (d). We discussed preference (e) above. With respect to preference (f), can this be known or even reliably predicted in advance?

Could it be reliably predicted that fewer of their preferences will be satisfied if they proceed with the pregnancy rather than opt for termination? This question leads on to several other more complex issues. In one sense Emma and her partner Elliot have already had a preference satisfied, namely for Emma to become pregnant. And also, if they choose to continue the pregnancy, a preference for Samuel to have a younger sibling would also have been satisfied. The news that the foetus has Down's syndrome causes them to revise their preferences.

The diagnosis of Down's syndrome prompts a drastic further refinement of preferences. As suggested above, this refinement is made against a background conception of what it is to lead a good life. If we accept preference satisfaction theory we might, straightforwardly, say that the refinement of preferences to have a child without a genetic anomaly now supersedes any previous related preference. But within preference satisfaction theory, in order to defeat certain objections to it (relating to perverse or highly objectionable preferences), it has been proposed that preferences can be 'laundered' (Goodin, 1986). One justification for such 'laundering' is that preferences may be based upon false information. The case of Emma Loach and her pregnancy may be just such a situation. Suppose we cast the preferences of Emma and her partner in the following way: they desire another child, a sibling for Samuel, and a good life (however this is construed).

Their having a Down's syndrome child is not incompatible with their leading a good life, even as this is construed within preference satisfaction theory. For they may still attain a *threshold* of satisfied preferences even with a child with Down's syndrome. Could it be shown their opportunities to lead a *maximally* good life are jeopardised by the birth of such a child? Such a proof would at least have to produce good grounds to support the conclusion that their opportunities for preference satisfaction are minimised. A difficulty with any attempt to provide such a case is that, of course, their preferences may change when they have the Down's syndrome child (*see* Reinders (2000) on this topic). Also, suppose the 'laundered preferences' strategy referred to above is permitted. If it is allowed that their overriding preference is to lead a good life, where this involves preferences for a fulfilling and rewarding family life, and a fulfilling career, again it is not at all clear that the presence of a Down's syndrome child will inevitably or even probably minimise opportunities to achieve this.

The domestic/public distinction, employed earlier, is also relevant here, for opportunities for preference satisfaction of all the family members may be maximised given sufficient support from the public sphere. As mentioned previously, this is an issue we will return to later, for plainly it impacts upon the preferences of the broader population since the availability of such resources will depend upon public taxation.

Before moving on to consider the third theory of the good life to be considered here, the most convincing reason in favour of termination in cases such as Emma Loach's, from the perspective of preference satisfaction theory, needs to be addressed. This is that, as far as the prospective Down's syndrome child is concerned, his likely short life expectancy implies that his opportunities for preference satisfaction are minimised. In other words, fewer life years means fewer opportunities for preference satisfaction.

As within our discussion of hedonistic theory, there are a number of ways of responding to this point. A first one is to say that a life span of 50–60 years is still quite a considerable one, if below average in modern western countries. Suppose Emma had been informed that her child would not have any genetic anomalies associated with disability, but would have a life expectancy of between 50 and 60 years. Would that have led her to terminate the pregnancy? Of course we do not know, but it is reasonable to conjecture she would have proceeded with the pregnancy. For a life with 50–60 years of satisfied preferences can still be a good life (again resorting to appeal to a threshold), even if it could have been better if longer.

Second, does this line generate absurd consequences? Suppose one was pregnant with twins, due to advances in genetic science it could reliably be predicted that one twin could expect to live for 80 years and two months and the other for 80 years, two months and one day. Surely it would be absurd to terminate the latter on the grounds that this affects their respective capacities to lead a good life. Yet adoption of the general principle 'always select for longer lives' seems to imply this would be defensible grounds for termination.

Third, most radically, it can be argued that the general principle 'more life years, more likelihood of leading a good life, due to greater availability of opportunities for preference satisfaction' is itself mistaken. Plainly this is an option available to those who do not subscribe to preference satisfaction theory. As will be seen, a proponent of the ideal or 'objective goods' theory could adopt such a strategy. Indeed, it should be acknowledged that preference satisfaction theory does appear vulnerable to some serious objections (to be rehearsed when we have considered all three theories).

Lastly, it should not be forgotten that more life years also present more opportunities for thwarting of preferences. One cannot assume that the additional capacity for preference satisfaction presented by extra life years, masks the additional capacity for preferences to be thwarted.

Overall, then, from the perspective of preference satisfaction theory we have seen that the most persuasive – if not compelling – ground for termination is that stemming from a 'maximising' view, in this case maximising of preference satisfaction. But we have provided a more than adequate rebuttal of such a ground.

A preference satisfaction theory of a good human life does not show that disability is always incompatible with leading a good life. Nor is it clear it shows that disablement makes leading a good life less likely (i.e. at least for those disabilities which do not obstruct the formulation of preferences). For the relationship between increased life years and increased preference satisfaction is a contingent one.

Having considered two of the main theories of the good life, let us now turn to the third: the 'ideal' or, equivalently, the 'objective goods' theory.

An 'objective goods' theory

There is a history of theories of the good life stretching back at least to Plato (*The Republic*) and Aristotle (*Nichomachean Ethics* (*NE*)). The main proposal here, obviously, is that a good human life consists in the attainment of certain objective goods. The Aristotelean theory has been an influential theory of this type, and has undergone something of a revival in recent years (*see* Nussbaum, 1988; Nussbaum and Sen, 1993). It is this particular example of an objective goods theory which will serve as our exemplar for this kind of approach to the question: 'what is a good life?'.

The Aristotelean conception of a good human life can be explained as follows. The key to answering the question of what is a good human life, from Aristotle's point of view is to ask, first, 'what is good in itself?', what is intrinsically good so to speak, as opposed to instrumentally good. And then second, to ask what the *function* of man is.

Translations of Aristotle's work tend to use the term 'man' in this context, as if the question of what is a good human life is synonymous with the question of what is a good life for man. I'll avoid such usage and, though it sounds slightly clumsy, speak of the good life for a human being, or a good human life.

Identification of the *unique* function of a human being discloses what the good life for humans will involve. Pursuit of the key function will be involved in pursuit of the good life.

The good that Aristotle identifies as being good in itself, intrinsically good, and thus as central to the good life, is that of flourishing, or living well, sometimes translated as 'happiness': 'happiness [flourishing] appears to be such an end' (*NE*, p.36). That is, it is aimed at not for instrumental reasons, in the way that, say, obtaining money may be aimed for. But is aimed at simply for its own sake. So a good human life aims at flourishing, or equivalently, living well.

Hence is it evident that the Aristotelean line conflicts radically with preference satisfaction theory, in that preferences are a means to an end (whatever satisfies them). So the approach may be criticised from the Aristotelean perspective for elevating instrumental goods (preferences) into intrinsic ones – regarding preferences as intrinsically good.

To turn now to the question of what the unique function of humans is, the key function which Aristotle identifies is that of rational activity. And crudely, engaging in this is a crucial component of what he considers to be a good human life. The steps taken to this conclusion are quite straightforward (if controversial). He reasons that the 'mere act of living' is not unique to humans, since – obviously – plants, worms and other creatures are alive. Therefore the unique function of humans, and the good life for them involves more than simply being alive (*NE*, p.38), e.g. in a vegetative state.

What of a 'life confined to experience of sensations' (*NE*, p.38)? But of course, nor is this unique to humans; it is shared by 'brute' animals – horses and cows etc. Therefore a good human life involves more than just the experience of sensations (and therefore, if we accept the Aristotelean line, the hedonistic theory must be mistaken).

Aristotle's conclusion is that the good life for a human involves reason and action 'good for man is an activity of the soul in accord with goodness' (i.e. right action) (*NE*, p.39). Hence, as mentioned above, although the exercise of rationality itself is a necessary component of the good life, it is not sufficient. Rationality must aim at virtue. So living well – flourishing – will involve using one's capacity for rationality in pursuit of virtue.

In addition, we are told that the good life 'cannot be achieved in less than a complete lifetime' (*NE*, p.39). This is confirmed in a memorable, if slightly misleading, expression: 'Call no man happy so long as he is alive' (*NE*, p.45). The point here is that one cannot judge a life to have been a good life until it has been completed.

To see this, consider the millionaire media tycoon Robert Maxwell. He seemed to have led a good life, by Aristotelean standards. He was successful in public and domestic life, was a philanthropist and fought for his country. For Aristotle, a good life is 'a fully rounded life' (*NE*, p.48), and Robert Maxwell certainly seems to have led one. After his death, however, very significant financial anomalies emerged in his business dealings, and many of his employees were deprived of pensions to which they were entitled, due directly to Maxwell's questionable use of pension funds for other purposes.

The point here is that, if a good life involves being a good person, as it seems to on the Aristotelean view (since one's acts must accord with goodness), due to the events which unfolded after Robert Maxwell's death, he could not be said to have lived a good life. It is in this way, then that 'call no man happy as long as he is alive' is true. Given that 'happy', strictly speaking, means something much more substantive, and would include 'morally good', we cannot say someone led a good life until their life is over. And even then, if certain facts came to light which showed the person concerned to have behaved in morally reprehensible ways, we may always revise a judgement to the effect that a person lived a good (or a bad) life.

So although the references to 'happiness' may suggest to us that Aristotle's line is close to the hedonistic theory, this is not the case. Aristotle's view is in fact clearly incompatible with the hedonistic view, since in that the mere experience of pleasure is sufficient to lead a good life. But as we saw above, a good life for a human must involve more than this for Aristotle.

As noted, the Aristotelean line also suggests preference satisfaction theory is inadequate. This is because people may have preferences that are not good for them and do not make it likely they will achieve a good life. The Robert Maxwell example appears to show this. Arguably, preferences to amass a personal fortune were given greater weight by him than the preferences to leave secure pensions for his employees. And people, for social reasons such as ideological oppression and indoctrination, may not consider some options, e.g. women and education in some developing countries (Sen, 1993). Here certain 'goods' may not occur to people as components of a good life because of the way they have been indoctrinated by a specific cultural ideology (Sen, 1993). In such cases their preferences are, thus, limited due to ideological constraints.

So we have given a brief outline of one specific 'objective goods' theory of the good life and have shown how the theory differs from hedonistic and preference satisfaction approaches. It should be made plain that the theory is still quite vague, though this does not need to concern us too much for our purposes. What matters is that the good life involves exercise of rationality and achievement of moral goods; in Aristotle's case these will be virtues such as courage, magnanimity, generosity and so on.

We need not agree with any specific list of such goods. All that matters for present purposes is understanding of the claim that a good life involves rationality in a way connected up to achievement of objective moral goods – or as Brock puts it: 'the realization of specific, explicitly normative ideals' (Brock, 1993, p.97).

Griffin, in his discussion, suggests 'accomplishment, deep personal relations, and the enjoyment of beauty' (Griffin, 1986, p.70) as examples of such objective goods. It should be stressed that none of these candidates for objective goods is being put forward here as sufficient for achieving a good life. Rather, all that is being done is to draw attention to the kinds of goods that may reasonably be judged to feature in a good life.

It is also worth noting that all the proposed candidate 'goods' offered thus far presuppose that the capacity for and exercise of autonomous choice is an important (perhaps even necessary) component of a good life. This does look like a plausible claim. To see this, ask whether we could credibly judge that a life shorn of such a capacity constitutes a good human life. Could it defensibly be maintained that a life in a permanent vegetative state (PVS) (from birth to death) is a good human life? It is surely very implausible to claim that it could be such. A similar story can be given in relation to the syndrome Z example. Not only is this a life shorn of autonomy, racked with pain, it is a life in which there is no capacity for moral sensitivity, nor accomplishment, nor appreciation of the aesthetic dimension of human life: the sight and sound of the sea, of birdsong, music, and so on.

And, in sympathy with the Aristotelean conception, it does seem plausible that a good life involves more than the exercise of rationality, no matter how impressive this capacity is within an individual. A good life, surely, involves moral sensitivity, the capacity to be moved by the plight of others for example. To see this, consider whether a supremely rational person would be said to have lived a good life if they showed no sense of moral sensitivity.

A further difference between Aristotle's objective goods theory and the previous two theories can be explained as follows. The previous two theories bind the criteria for leading a good life to what can be termed 'subjective' states. This is most obviously so in relation to the hedonistic theory. As we heard, the goodness or otherwise of a life is determined solely by the qualities of subjectively experienced mental states. The preference satisfaction theory can also be described as subjective, though in a different way. It is subjective in the sense that just what is preferred (the content of the preferences) is left to each individual to decide.

Consider now then the various parties we have been considering in relation to this theory of the good life. First let us focus on Emma Loach's prospective son. We know that Down's syndrome is compatible with possession of the capacity for rationality. A significant proportion of people with Down's syndrome have this capacity. As we heard, on the Aristotelean conception of a good life, this capacity has to be married to the capacity for moral sensitivity and judgement. The question of whether a person has such a capacity is in many ways difficult to resolve. But minimally it must involve some sense of moral rightness and wrongness, in addition to moral sensitivity (this can be defined in terms of a concern for the plight of others which is not motivated solely by self-interest). Some of the attributes mentioned by Griffin also sound relevant: 'accomplishment, deep personal relations, and the enjoyment of beauty' (Griffin, 1986, p.70).

It is reasonable to assume that at least a significant number of people with Down's syndrome possess the capacities highlighted so far. But decisions to terminate pregnancy will inevitably be based upon statistical probabilities. So even if it is said that one or two people with Down's syndrome have the capacity to lead a good life, prospective parents will want to know how likely it is that their child will have that capacity. As before, though, it is my contention that it is important to signal the fact that there is no incompatibility between Down's syndrome (and other disabling conditions) and capacity to pursue a good life, for the opposite is often assumed.

Returning to the question of the proportion of people with Down's syndrome that possess the capacity to lead a good life, this will be cashed out as follows. How many have the capacities for rationality and moral sensitivity and judgement, and for any other of the capacities deemed necessary for being able to lead a good life, e.g. accomplishment, aesthetic appreciation etc? Answering these questions would be an empirical task, not one we can undertake here. But it does not seem unlikely that research into these questions would find many instances of people with Down's syndrome (perhaps the majority of such people) who do possess such capacities. And, looking further afield, it is plain that very significant proportions of people with other disabling conditions also possess such capacities (Murphy, 1987; Oliver, 1990; Morris, 1991; Toombs, 1995; and so on). If so, then, two familiar claims can be advanced. First, Down's syndrome and other disabling conditions (excepting conditions such as syndrome Z) are not incompatible with possession of the capacities necessary for leading a good human life, as this is understood within an objective goods theory. Second, it is not even clear that Down's syndrome or other conditions make attainment of a good human life less likely. For such conditions provide scope for accomplishment, exercise of rationality, and moral sensitivity and judgement.

What of Samuel, Emma's existing son? He plainly has the capacity to lead a good life even with a younger sibling who has Down's syndrome. So there is no question of any incompatibility between capacity to lead a good life and having a brother with Down's syndrome. But can he lead a maximally good life, by the lights of an objective goods theory? It is not clear to me that Samuel's prospects are hampered by the birth of the sibling with Down's syndrome. His capacities for moral sensitivity and rationality need not be impugned. Nor need there be obstacles toward accomplishments and deep personal relations.

Turn now to Emma and her partner Elliot. There is no doubting they have the capacity to pursue a good life in the light of the theory we are currently considering. It follows there is no incompatibility between their giving birth to a Down's syndrome child and leading a good life. Arguably, their capacity for accomplishment and moral sympathy may be enhanced by the presence of a Down's syndrome child within the family. Reinders' work suggests that such familial experiences generate opportunities for 'moral growth'. Reinders develops what he terms an 'enrichment claim' (Reinders, 2000, pp.166–8). Drawing upon accounts written by parents of disabled children, he proposes that there are certain goods that are only achievable by engaging in a struggle. They include the kinds of goods sought and achieved by successful athletes. But also, he suggests, such goods can be achieved by the process of raising children with disabilities.

One implication of this line of argument is that the capacity for Emma Loach and her partner for leading a good life may, in fact, be enhanced by having a child with Down's syndrome. So, controversially, it may be claimed that capacity to lead a good life is enhanced by the presence of a disabled person within the family.

Against this, it may be argued as follows. Opportunities to spend time with the existing sibling Samuel may be reduced and so – assuming being a good parent is also an element of the good life – Emma and Elliot are less good parents to Samuel because of the presence of the child with Down's syndrome. Similarly, it could be claimed that Emma and Elliot have fewer career opportunities due to the time they need to devote to caring for their disabled child. So, if a good life does indeed include accomplishments, and if a successful career is regarded as a significant accomplishment, then Emma's life, and that of her partner, may well be less good than it could have been. In other words, although the capacity for Emma and partner Elliot to lead a good life is not impugned if we apply a 'threshold' standard, it may be impugned if we hold a maximising one.

In partial response to the last point, it is here again that matters of distributive justice emerge. For if there are sufficient levels of social support, the couples' capacity to pursue a career and spend time with their existing son need not be jeopardised.

These questions of distributive justice raise very large questions about the kind of society citizens would like to live in. Is it one which provides the kind of support which *may* be needed by disabled people? In her discussion of the good state or society, Nussbaum (1988) draws upon Aristotle's work on this topic. Her conclusion is that a good society by Aristotelian lights (and by hers) is one which provides the conditions within which its citizens can lead a good life. Of course this extends to all its citizens. This is an attractive proposal to many, it does not of course ensure that all citizens will lead a good life, but it is one where those with the capacity to do so can flourish.

Adoption of such a policy would rule out individuals who do not have the capacity to flourish – e.g. those with syndrome Z. But it would entail that those with the capacity to flourish could expect the conditions to be in place to enable them to do so. So in this kind of Aristotelian state, Emma's family could expect the conditions to be in place to enable them to lead a good life. So too could anyone with Down's syndrome, assuming it is typically the case that people with Down's syndrome possess the capacities to lead a good life by Aristotelian standards (capacities for rationality, moral sensitivity and judgement). Of course the provision of such resources is controversial and likely to come from general taxation. And some may object to contributing to others' wellbeing more than they are required to at present. Others might not object of course. As mentioned, these issues raise the question of the kind of society people should live in. As seen, the Aristotelean answer is one which creates the conditions for its citizens to pursue a good life. Others may object that this would impinge too much on their capacity to pursue a good life, for example if they are required to pay high levels of taxation.

In a recent article in a UK newspaper, Jane Campbell (2003) describes herself as follows:

> I was born with spinal muscular atrophy, a so-called 'terminal' condition. I cannot lift my head from the pillow unaided and I need a ventilator to help me breathe at night … I have a high-powered and fulfilling job as the head of a major national organisation. More importantly, I am fortunate to live in a borough that provides exemplary social care: a 24-hour personal assistant enables me to have an independent life, to be a wife to my husband and a person to my family and friends (Campbell, 2003, p.1).

The relevance of this article should be plain. The likely response to the points made above concerning Aristotle's idea of a good society is that decisions such as that taken by Emma Loach and Elliot occur in today's context, not in an Aristotelian one. So if her child were to need social support, could she expect it? According to this article, she may well be able to expect it.

The key question, from a philosophical perspective, though, is whether she is entitled to expect such levels of support. The support is funded from general taxation. So, strictly speaking, other people are paying to sustain Jane Campbell's quality of life – though she too is a tax payer of course.

This book is not a book on political philosophy, and the question of whether Jane Campbell and other disabled people are entitled to receive extensive public support hinges upon questions within the sphere of political philosophy, specifically, on the question of the nature of the political state. It may be useful to simply review quickly some main options when it comes to the question of what counts as a just society.

One extreme position is that one is entitled to keep what one has and what one earns (Nozick, 1974), and one is only obliged to pay taxation to sustain a minimal state. Broadly speaking, this will include only emergency services and security services. On this view, education and health are matters for each individual. As individuals we can choose to spend money on these – for ourselves or for our children – or choose not to. We are not obliged to pay for the health or education of others however. Of course we may *choose* to do so, but we cannot justly be compelled to do so – as tax-paying citizens of contemporary liberal democracies are currently so compelled.

Clearly if a view of this kind prevailed, Emma could not assume that support funded by the 'public sphere' will be available, should her prospective child need such support. And hence the prospects for all involved for leading a good life may be significantly impugned.

A second view at least implies that a just society is one in which vulnerable members will be supported. This view, derivable from the work of Rawls (1970), invites us to imagine a group of potential citizens deliberating upon the question of what is a fair society. They are to do this behind a veil of ignorance, hence they do not know whether they will be rich, poor, talented, untalented or whatever. Rawls concludes that, due to adoption of enlightened self-interest, such people will 'play safe' and ensure that social arrangements are such that the worst off still have a reasonable standard of living. This idea approximates the Aristotelean one mentioned above in which the ideal society is one which provides the conditions within which citizens with the capacity to flourish, to lead a good life, can do so. A society organised along these lines seems to hold out greater likelihood of creating conditions for its citizens to lead a good life, even by Aristotelean standards.

A third, communitarian, view is much closer to the second, Rawlsian, position but is importantly different. In the Rawlsian line, the nature of the just society stems from the participants' reasoning within a framework of 'enlightened self-interest'. So self-interest plays a key role, and the presumption is that this best captures the moral psychology of human beings. However, proponents of a third view point to societies such as those within Scandinavia and also in The Netherlands. Here it is said, citizens are bound together by feelings of 'solidarity'. This is a difficult idea to spell out clearly but is said to go beyond wishing to support fellow citizens merely out of self-interest, e.g. thinking that one should support vulnerable others merely because one may become vulnerable oneself. So here the idea is that one should offer moral support to fellow citizens simply because they are fellow citizens, and that a good society is one in which citizens care about the plight of one another and try to help those in need of help and support (for more on this view, *see* Munhall and Swift, 1992).

Of these three positions it is of course less likely that people such as Emma Loach could anticipate support from the public sphere given the Nozickian view. But the remaining two positions provide some scope for optimism, though of course it is impossible to specify how much support will be provided. This quick excursion into political philosophy does help to show that the assumption of 'lack of support' is not inevitably warranted. It is warranted only in a society organised along Nozickian lines.

Interestingly, the leader of the main UK opposition party, the Conservatives, recently issued a statement of 'core beliefs'. These include the belief that 'people must have every opportunity to fulfil their potential' (*Guardian* Homepage, 2 January 2004, p.1, www.guardian.co.uk). This expresses commitment to a view much closer to the Aristotelean society rather than the Nozickian one, and stems from a party whose views are often represented as closer to the latter and not the former.

Given our discussion of this last theory of the good life then, it seems reasonable to conclude once again that Emma's prospective child has the capacity to lead a good life, and that his prospects for leading a maximally good life need not be impugned. I would like to close this part of the discussion by tackling the 'maximising' view head on, and trying to show how it is a mistaken approach to adopt.

A critique of 'maximising' approaches to the question of capacity to lead a good life

As repeatedly mentioned above, one of the main considerations for termination when disability is diagnosed stems from the 'maximising' presupposition, namely that giving birth to a disabled child impugns that child's capacity to lead a maximally good life. It is time to subject that presupposition to some sustained critical scrutiny, as opposed to the skirmishes undertaken so far.

To rehearse the difference between 'threshold' and 'maximising' approaches to the question of whether disablement impugns a person's capacity to lead a good life (directly or indirectly). In the threshold approach it is presumed that one is capable of leading a good human life if one can undergo sufficient, pleasurable experiences, or have a sufficient number of preferences satisfied, or attain a sufficient quantity of objective goods. As in our discussion of hedonistic theory, difficulties were identified in trying to specify a threshold in advance.

In the threshold approach one asks 'Could my child have lead a good human life with this disabling trait?'. But on the 'maximising' approach one asks whether the disabling trait would impugn, in some way, the child's capacity to maximise those aspects of life that make for a good human life. Adoption of this approach may lead a prospective parent to ask: 'Would this genetic anomaly inhibit the capacity of my child to lead a maximally good human life?'. What constitutes 'maximally good' will obviously depend upon which theory of the good life one adopts.[3]

I think the distinction between maximising and threshold approaches is helpful since it explains in part some of the 'talking past' each other that occurs between bioethicists and some people with disabilities. The bioethicists make their points employing a 'maximising' conception of a good life. Some people with disabilities, in responding to these points, take the bioethicists to be stating that it

---

[3]Thus in discussion of this topic by Hare (1974), the issue is described as follows. Suppose one has a choice between (a) having a child now which lacks the capacity to undergo certain experiences (e.g. sensory ones) and (b) having a later child which does not lack the capacity to undergo them. Since having the capacity to undergo as wide a range of experiences as possible is a good thing (on the maximising view), one ought to have the later child since she has more avenues open to her to lead a good life.

is not possible to lead a good human life with a disability. They maintain that it is indeed possible to lead such a life while having a disability. But of course this view (that of the disabled people making these responses) employs the 'threshold' conception of what is involved in leading a good life rather than a maximising view (*see* Johnson, 2003).

Bioethicists who argue from a 'maximising' perspective can quite legitimately allow that a person with a disability can lead a good human life. But from the 'maximising' perspective, it is one which could have been even better if the person had not been disabled. It could have been better because more preferences could have been satisfied, more pleasurable experiences had, or more objective goods attained.

The maximising view is well represented in the following passage from Peter Singer:

> In general it does seem that the more highly developed the conscious life of the being, the greater the degree of self-aware-ness and rationality and the broader the range of possible experiences, the more one would prefer that kind of life, if one were choosing between it and a being at a lower level of awareness (Singer, 1993, p.107).

This quote from Singer expresses the maximising view very clearly. The greater the level of consciousness, the greater the degree of self-awareness, the greater the degree of rationality, the greater the range of possible experiences (e.g. sensory experiences), then the more preferable the life. 'More preferable' here is equivalent to 'the better the life', or more clumsily, 'the more good the life'.

Two main ways of responding to the maximising view are: first, to claim that disabling traits need not inhibit maximising; and second, to provide a radical challenge to the maximising view.

First response: disabling traits need not inhibit maximising

A proponent of the maximising strategy is likely to point to geneti-cally caused sensory disabilities as examples of disabilities in which the capacity to maximise is jeopardised (Singer, 1993; Harris, 2000).

In such cases the capacity to lead a maximally good life is thought to be jeopardised by factors tied to the physical constitution of the person. So consider this 'constitutional' restriction view in relation to the three theories.

With regard to the hedonistic theory a person with a severe sensory disability will not be capable of undergoing a specific range of pleasurable experiences, e.g. those that derive from the senses of sight or hearing.

But in response, it could be said that the absence of one sense has an intensifying effect on other sensory experiences. So although one kind of experience is closed to the individual, the intensity of other kinds of sensory experiences is enhanced. Thus a visually impaired person may say their senses of touch and hearing are intensified as a consequence of living without sight (*see* e.g. Sacks, 1995 in which he describes Virgil, a blind person, as 'a touch person through and through', p.132).

Also, one could ask why a life with a wide range of experiences open to one is better than a life with a narrower range of pleasurable experiences open to one. In the hedonistic theory, what matters is that one experiences as many pleasurable experiences as possible. It is not clear why a life in which one has intense pleasurable experiences via four routes gives fewer opportunities for pleasurable experiences than a life in which a person has five sensory routes via which to undergo pleasurable experiences.

We've been focusing on sensory disability so far in this part of the discussion but it is worth mentioning Down's syndrome in this context. It could be claimed that this actually maximises one's capacity for pleasurable experiences since it is associated with a pleasant, cheerful disposition. Minimally, it is not clear why moderate intellectual disability would impugn a person's capacity to undergo maximal pleasurable experiences, except in so far as it is associated with a shorter than average life span.

With regard to preference satisfaction theories, focusing again on severe sensory impairment, as seen, the 'maximiser' proposes that the sensory impairment entails that a range of preferences cannot be satisfied, and, hence, cannot be maximised.

But a preference satisfaction theorist is not entitled to make a claim of that kind. For as mentioned above, that theory cannot dictate the *types* of preferences a person should seek to satisfy on pain of lapsing into an 'objective goods' theory of the good life. So the only scope for a preference satisfaction theorist here is to argue that sensory disabilities inhibit capacity for maximal preference satisfaction. But it is not clear to me that this can be shown since the question of which preferences a person wishes to satisfy is an individual matter.

Moving on to intellectual disabilities, certain preferences might not be formulated, e.g. relating to complex intellectual activities, though, as seen above, this can be contested. 'Complexity' is a relative concept. What some find simple, others find complex. It could be said that a person with Down's syndrome can experience the intellectual pleasures of solving intellectual problems, but these are problems which others might not find so complex.

Also, other preferences will still be formulated, such as those for certain pleasurable experiences and maintenance of relationships with family and friends. So without specifying that some kinds of preferences are of intrinsic value it is hard again to see how a preference satisfaction theorist can argue that moderate intellectual disability inhibits the capacity to maximise preference satisfaction.

With regard to objective good theories, let us first agree on some likely candidates for these: achievement, happiness, flourishing, moral sensitivity, personal relationships. These presuppose within the individual the capacity for autonomy.

When viewed from the 'maximising' approach, the way in which disabilities fail to maximise achievement of these, presumably, is as follows. Sensory disabilities will obstruct the achievement of objective goods by virtue of their effects upon autonomy of action. So too will physical disabilities which affect mobility. Intellectual disabilities will limit an individual's capacity to attain the objective goods.

However, of course all these claims can be challenged. Controversially, it may be said that adversity maximises opportunities for achievement. But less controversially it is not clear how disability inhibits opportunities to develop the other objective goods just listed. Alderson observes that there is little research conducted on the quality of life of disabled people which asks disabled people themselves about their lives (Alderson, 2001). Indeed, this is the message behind the disability rights slogan 'Nothing about us without us'. As may be anticipated, Alderson tries to rectify this situation in her own work. In interviews she conducts with people with Down's syndrome, it is evident that the lives of the subjects she met involve attainment of the objective goods identified above – accomplishment, moral sensitivity, deep personal relationships and so on. Moreover, she echoes the point made above that the practice of prenatal screening for Down's syndrome itself has a negative impact upon the lives of people with that condition. As she points out, there is a bitter irony in this since there is no evidence to show such screening to be cost-effective, or to reduce suffering (this in an era in which 'evidence-based medicine' is lauded).

Let us turn now to a more radical response to the maximising view.

Second response: radical challenge to the maximising view

The points so far have been attempts to show that disablement is compatible with even the 'maximising' approach to the question of what is involved in a good human life. What I would like to move on to now is to present a radical challenge to the 'maximising view'.

Recall the quote from Peter Singer:

> In general it does seem that the more highly developed the conscious life of the being, the greater the degree of self-aware-ness and rationality and the broader the range of possible experiences, the more one would prefer that kind of life, if one were choosing between it and a being at a lower level of awareness (Singer, 1993, p.107).

To break this down a little, let us focus on the claims made about rationality, and about the broad range of possible experiences.

As noted earlier Singer seems to say here that the greater one's capacity for rationality, the more preferable one's life. But should this be accepted? Think of the way the 'super-intelligent' Mr Spock is occasionally lampooned in the TV show 'Star Trek'. It could be argued that Spock is not capable of leading a good human life because his powerful capacity for rationality is not tempered with qualities such as moral sensitivity and sympathy.

Also of course, one may well use a maximally developed capacity for rationality for morally good ends, but one may use the capacity for execution of evil acts too. Plainly it is possible to divorce means from ends here, that is, to divorce the capacity to attain an end (maximal rationality) from evaluation of the end achieved (is the act good or evil?). So the maximising view seems susceptible to the criticism that it mistakes means for ends. Having a highly developed capacity for rationality is not sufficient for leading a good life, it can be argued. What really matters are the ends to which this capacity is directed. This criticism draws attention to the erroneous emphasis on *means* within the maximising approach. Questions regarding what counts as a good life are more plausibly directed at *ends*.

So, possession of a maximal capacity for rationality may not be a sufficient condition for leading a good human life. Nor is it a necessary condition, as our discussion above shows (e.g. with reference to people with moderate intellectual disabilities).

With regard to the 'broader the range of possible experiences' mentioned in the quote, the suggestion here is that the greater one's capacity for 'possible experiences' the more preferable – the better – one's life. But again, should this be accepted?

Paul Churchland raises the hypothetical case of a race of beings capable of visually seeing temperature (Churchland, 1979, p.8). They have open to them a range of visual experiences not open to humans. The 'maximising' approach adopted by Singer seems to imply that a life with that additional perceptual faculty is preferable to one with only the sensory faculties typically available to humans – sight, hearing, touch, taste, smell. But is this really the case? Would a life with more avenues for sensory experience be a better human life than one with fewer; better *solely* for that reason (assuming the usual five sensory faculties are present too).

One can imagine situations in which the capacity to see temperature would come in handy. One could select the coolest can of beer from the fridge since one could see which was the coolest. Or one could avoid a bad burn by seeing that a surface is extremely hot though it appears normal to a person without the facility to see temperature. So there are circumstances in which this imagined faculty may be of use and may make one's life go better.[4]

But, if anything, this point reinforces the view that such a faculty is a mere instrument. The question of whether or not one lived a good life just does seem separable from the question of how many sensory faculties one has. For, surely, as an objective good theory serves to remind us, it is ends which are of greater importance in a human life, more so than means.

---

[4]I'm indebted to Stephen Wilkinson for pointing this out.

Also, it sounds absurd to claim that the more senses one has the greater one's chances of leading a good life, so that a life with 31 sensory channels is a better one than a life with 30. Yet the maximising approach requires acceptance of such a view. In fact one might point out that the more sensory data one receives the more difficult they are to process, and so overall cognitive competence declines.

In the quote above, Singer mistakenly accords greatest weight to what are, after all, instrumental rather than intrinsic goods. And, as in Aristotle's discussion of the good life, it seems reasonable to regard the good life as being bound up with intrinsic and not instrumental goods. Thus rationality is good since it helps us accomplish certain ends. But it is the ends which are of ultimate value, not the means by which we attain them.

So we have good reasons to reject the maximising approach. It focuses on means and neglects ends. It is achievement of ends which makes a life a good life. What would need to be shown is that disability compromises a person's chances for leading a good life, where this involves attainment of objective goods (given that a hedonistic view is implausible). But setting aside conditions such as syndrome Z, it is not clear that this can be shown. Disability need not compromise an individual's capacity for a life involving moral sensitivity, aesthetic appreciation, deep relationships and accomplishment.

Also, in further opposition to the maximising view in all cases, the question of whether or not a person led a good life is answered by reference to a threshold perspective on this question. As we saw, this is the meaning behind a question pondered over by Aristotle; namely the question of whether we should 'call no man happy so long as he is alive' (*NE*, p.45). The answer to this given above was indeed that – given a much richer conception of happiness – one cannot judge a life to have been a good one until it is over, until the facts are known, so to speak. The making of such judgements inescapably invokes a threshold. So actual judgements invoke this rather than a maximising life. A life can still be a good life even though one may be able to pose the question 'Could it have been better?'.

Let us finally return to the case of Emma Loach. Does this discussion cast any light on her predicament? It is the case that her decision is informed, if only tacitly, by conceptions of a good life. I think enough has been said here to warrant acceptance of that claim. The conclusions regarding the discussion of the three theories of the good life led to a rejection of the maximising view. So the key question is whether or not a possibly disabling impairment impugns a person's capacity to lead a good life, where this means to attain objective goods. If one can confidently answer 'yes' to this question, then termination seems justified. Otherwise it seems harder to justify.

Finally, let us not forget also the problem of defining disability in the first place. As we saw, this cannot always be 'read off' from physical characteristics (impairments).

Conclusion

As seen in our discussion in this part, none of the three theories of a good life show life with disablement to be incompatible with leading a good human life. Nor is it clear that disability always makes leading a good human life less likely – even when compared against all three theories of what counts as such a life.

Our discussion has focused on some of the ethical considerations raised by the practice of termination of pregnancy on grounds of disabling traits within the foetus. It has been maintained that such decisions presuppose a conception of what is a good human life. It has been argued that a life with disability is not always incompatible with leading such a life. Nor need disability always impair the prospects for leading a good human life. These conclusions have been reached following consideration of three main philosophical theories of what a good human life consists of.

The point of the 'syndrome Z' example was to try to give an example of a condition which appears incompatible with leading a good human life. So here the very *capacity* to lead such a life is jeopardised due to the nature of the syndrome. However, many disabilities are not as debilitating as syndrome Z and need not impugn the capacity of an individual to lead a good human life. In such disabilities there will be only a contingent relationship – and not a necessary one – between possession of the relevant disabling genetic trait and inability of the person to lead a good human life. That 'inability' will be due to factors beyond the person with the disabling trait and not (wholly) due to factors intrinsic to the person.

Here I fall back on the earlier excursion into political philosophy. The Rawlsian and Communitarian societies seem more likely to make such changes to the social environment than the Nozickian one. And we should bear in mind the point about the Aristotelian society; this will be one which creates conditions intended to facilitate the flourishing of its citizens. Given this, one could expect the social environment to be shaped to be consistent with that aim.

We turn next to a discussion of the relationship between disablement and the person. As will be seen, the account of the person endorsed in the discussion lends further weight to the theory of disablement supported in Part One.

PART THREE

Disablement and the person

Introduction

In this, Part Three of our discussion, we will look at the relationship between disablement and the person, and also disablement and identity. We will begin by showing how differing philosophical conceptions of the person have importantly different implications for the way disablement is conceived of. Differing ontologies of the person imply differing conceptions of disablement. And differing ontologies of the person also motivate differing views of disablement when this is viewed from a moral perspective. (By differing 'ontologies of the person' it is meant different views on the nature of persons: are they wholly physical; part physical, part mental; wholly mental; spiritual?)

We then turn to look at the relationship between disabling characteristics and the identities of persons. A number of commentators claim their disability to be a part of their identity (Murphy, 1987; Oliver, 1990; Morris, 1991; Toombs, 1995, p.12; also *see* Sacks, 1995, p.278). Oliver, for example, is explicit that 'disability is an essential part of the self' (Oliver, 1990, p.xiii), not 'detachable' or separable from the person.

An attempt to assess such claims will need to address the general question: 'What are the kinds of properties which serve to identify particular persons, what is it that sustains a person's identity over time?'. One option is to view disablement as a contingent property of a person, not something central in any deep sense to their personal identity. But according to a rival view, such as that expressed by Oliver, disablement can be 'essential' to the identity of the person, a characteristic fundamental to their personal identity.

The question of the relationship between disability and identity is further prompted by consideration of a response to the practice of prenatal genetic diagnosis (PGD) from a 'disability rights' perspective. As will be seen, some groups of disabled people hold the view that PGD sends a message to the effect that it would have been better if they had not been born.

Thus consider a person currently living with cystic fibrosis. Such a person might hold the view that PGD of cystic fibrosis implies that it would have been better had he not been born.

Last but not least, the question of the relationship between disablement and identity is of intrinsic interest. The problem of personal identity is a long-standing philosophical problem which, in the eyes of many, has never been satisfactorily resolved. It may be that by looking at the problem from a disablement perspective, unexpected progress can be made.

Three philosophical theories of the person, and their implications for disablement

Oversimplifying greatly, but not misleadingly, it is reasonable to claim that there are three main philosophical theories concerning the nature of human persons. The first holds that they are composed of two kinds of substance, mind and body. Of these it is mind which is central – essential – to their nature. For obvious reasons, this is described as a *dualist* view, and it is associated with the philosopher Descartes (1637, 1641, 1649).

According to a second view, humans are wholly physical things (Smart, 1959; Wilson, 1979). For obvious reasons we can describe this as a *physicalist* view. So there is no separable 'mind substance', only physical matter.

A third view is one we can term *emergentism* (*see* e.g. Broad, 1929; McGinn, 1982, pp.30–1). This agrees with physicalism in allowing that humans are composed of physical matter, but it holds that when their physical parts reach a certain level of sophisticated organisation, other properties emerge. Such properties include consciousness, mental life, thoughts, feelings etc.

We will return to discuss emergentism later, for now, however, we will look in more detail at the dualist view. This has been extremely influential in informing understandings of disablement, and in generating a particular, individualistic, conception of the person which has some negative moral implications for disabled people.

Cartesian dualism and disablement

As mentioned, this generates specific conceptions of disablement, and of the nature of persons with disabilities, such that they cannot be 'legitimate persons' in a sense to be made clear shortly.

The Cartesian heritage fosters a model of physical disablement according to which the self is left 'intact' or whole, since the mind is purportedly unaffected by physical disability. According to this conception: a self is encased, housed, or trapped within a body (Murphy writes 'Hey, it's the same old me inside this body', 1987, p.70). The boxer Muhammad Ali was once described as being 'housed' within a body wracked by Parkinson's disease (*The Observer*, 2 March 1997). Time and again one encounters such claims regarding physical disablement. As Murphy suggests, it is as if the mind remains as it has always been, but it is now trapped, housed etc within a body it can no longer control.

It is also part of this Cartesian heritage that the mental and physical realms, are clearly demarcated. Thus phenomena are either mental, or physical, not both. And it is also part of this overall picture that the human body is an object different from inanimate objects only by virtue of the degree of complexity of its organisation. In disablement, the implication is that the instructions issued by the 'intact' person, cannot be properly followed due to a mechanical failure of the machine.

The Cartesian conception applies less straightforwardly in the case of intellectual and sensory disabilities. But, nonetheless, it can be applied. The conception of intellectual disability fostered by the Cartesian view is a mirror-image of that of physical disability. Instead of an 'intact' self encased within a body which does not function properly, a view is fostered of an intact body capable of full function were the self able to instruct it properly (witness the title of Burt's book *The Subnormal Mind* (Burt, 1937)).

With reference to sensory disabilities, the Cartesian position generates a view such that a type of sensory information typically available to persons is not available to the person with a sensory impairment. As with physical disabilities, the Cartesian line suggests a person, although deprived of a range of information (such as vision or sound), remains an 'intact' person. So the restoration or introduction of the relevant range of sensory information has no substantial effect on the person. All that occurs is that the person is now furnished

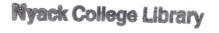

with a range of information previously unavailable to it. As Sacks puts it: 'This is the commonsensical notion – that the eyes will be opened ... the blind man will "receive" sight' (Sacks, 1995, p.103).

Thus, the above comments express support for the claim that disability is commonly conceived of in broadly Cartesian terms. This applies most straightforwardly to physical disability, but can be carried over to motivate conceptions of intellectual and sensory disabilities.

Cartesian dualism and individualism

As mentioned above, Cartesian presuppositions imply that people with disabilities are somehow illegitimate persons, are deeply flawed in some sense. This is because the Cartesian view is one in which the person is held to be a being that is wholly *independent*. Independence is part of the very nature, the essence, of the person: as Descartes writes: 'I [am] a substance whose whole essence or nature is to be conscious and whose being requires no place and depends upon no material thing' (Descartes, 1637, p.32).

This philosophical conception of persons is sometimes described as individualistic in nature. It is individualistic in the sense that the existence of the person is held to be wholly independent of any other thing (for Descartes, strictly speaking, apart from God). Its existence owes nothing to anything outside itself, nor does its nature, that is, the particular character or set of mental characteristics exhibited by the person. So on this Cartesian view of what it is to be a person, the person could potentially exist independently of any set of social arrangements, and independently of any cultural conventions or linguistic forms.

According to this form of individualism a 'legitimate person' so to speak, is one who owes their existence and individuality to no other thing. What makes you you, the characteristics that make you the person you are, are determined by characteristics entirely within you. According to this picture of the human person, a legitimate self is an ontologically independent self, one which owes its existence and identity to no other thing.

This form of individualism (ontological individualism), directly inspired by the Cartesian view of the person, generates a certain position in morality too. This position asserts the primacy of the wishes of the individual. It is described by Lukes as 'ethical individualism' (Lukes, 1973, pp.99–106). In this, the ideal person is conceived as one who is fully autonomous, able to make her own choices concerning how she wants to lead her own life. In elaboration of the characteristics of the 'ideal' liberal individual, Gauthier (1986) identifies three key features: (a) 'First of all the liberal individual is an active being ...' (p.153); (b) 'Second, the liberal individual has her own independent conception of the good' (p.154); (c) and third 'the liberal individual is fully rational, where rationality embraces both autonomy and the capacity to choose' (p.154). This form of liberalism stems directly from the position Lukes labels ethical individualism.

It is worth stressing just how prominently the characteristic of *independence* is emphasised within both ontological individualism, and the kind of ethical individualism just outlined. According to ontological individualism a person is, by definition, ontologically independent. According to normative individualism a person is an independent thinker, fully rational and active. Murphy again states: 'Independence, self-reliance and autonomy are central values in American culture' (Murphy, 1987, p.154).

In light of wide acceptance of a Cartesian conception of the person it is not surprising that disability is considered to be a 'bad thing'. For disability – correctly or incorrectly – is often characterised in terms of dependence upon others (*see* e.g. Heaton-Ward and Wiley, 1984, p.21; Oliver, 1993). Thus we have a philosophical picture, generated by Cartesianism, of the 'ideal' person as an independent person. But in many people's minds disability is defined in terms of its entailing dependence. Hence, if a philosophy of individualism is widespread we should not be surprised that disability is considered to be a bad thing.

This seems especially to be the case when intellectual disability is considered. The individualist line stresses independence and the intellectual capacity needed to be an autonomous individual. Yet these characteristics are compromised in intellectual disablement, thus impugning the legitimacy of the intellectually disabled person: such a person lacks independence and autonomy, two key values in the individualist ethos.

There are various ways of responding to this situation. Suppose the basic tenets of Cartesian-inspired individualism are accepted; that is, suppose the ontological and ethical presumptions of individualism are correct. Focus on the ethical aspects. As we saw in Part One, proponents of a social model of disablement argue (Oliver, 1990) that many people with disabilities, especially physical disabilities, do in fact have the capacity to match the characteristics of the ideal liberal individual. It is just that social factors such as the poor wheelchair accessibility of public buildings and transport conspire to prevent disabled people from manifesting their capacity for independent thought and activity.

In a memorable, if depressing, image the front cover of Oliver's (1990) book is a picture of a man in a wheelchair at the foot of a flight of steps. The steps are the only entrance to a polling station. The picture dramatically makes Oliver's point. People with disabilities are perfectly capable of matching the characteristics of the ideal liberal individual, if only certain problems of accessibility to public facilities and institutions are forthcoming. The implication here is that the individualistic conception of the person need not generate negative implications about life with disability, or for disabled people, providing certain social changes are made. Those with 'intact' minds but impaired bodies, it seems, can still play the role of the 'ideal' liberal individual. (It is interesting to see how such Cartesian modes of thinking of disablement persist in the present day, as is the case, arguably, with the social model.)

It should be pointed out that this response – modifying the social environment – leaves untouched the philosophical views which motivate individualism. Hence it goes only a very limited way towards addressing the challenge posed by individualism to disabled persons. The response works best when we have in mind people who have disabilities that affect their mobility. But how does it generalise over to apply to intellectually disabled people, or people with serious sensory disabilities? It appears not to. Social changes will not restore sight to a person unable to see, or significantly increase the cognitive capacity of a very severely intellectually disabled person.

As we have just seen, the response generated by the social model seeks to show how disability need not impede pursuance of the ideal life as this is understood within ethical individualism. A different way of responding is to call into question the basic tenets of both ontological and ethical individualism.

With regard to ontological individualism, a credible way to challenge this is to reject the Cartesian view of the person it adheres to. The first way of criticising it is to focus attention on the way it appears completely to sever the mental and physical realms. As traditionally understood, the Cartesian position is that these realms are in fact separable (Descartes states: 'I am really distinct from my body and could exist without it' (1641/1954, p.115, sixth meditation)). This seems quite an extravagant ontological claim given overwhelming amounts of empirical data which suggest that mental phenomena require the presence of some underlying physical phenomena (a nervous system or computer hardware or some other physical substrate).

There are other difficulties for the Cartesian position, of which Descartes was aware, concerning causation between the two realms. How can this occur given their radically different natures? (Though it should be acknowledged that this is a problem for the other two theories also, in differing ways.)

There is an enormous amount of literature on this topic and it is not appropriate to rehearse the merits and problems of Cartesian dualism further here (*see* e.g. Williams, 1978; McGinn, 1982). But there is another criticism, related to questions of personal identity to be advanced later which can also be drawn upon now. (Such questions concern what it is that makes us the same person, over periods of time.)

As noted, the Cartesian position asserts the independence of the person to such an extent that even the very identity of the person can be articulated without the need to appeal to phenomena outside the mind of the person. But is this a credible line to take? One might plausibly point to the extent to which the identities of persons are determined by factors beyond their bodies or minds. Indeed, this is a view we will discuss further below. It can be argued that the identities of persons are at least in part determined by what is most important to them: their moral projects, their relationships, their work and so on. Moreover, it is argued, that instead of persons being considered essentially individualistic, independent beings, they are in fact essentially dependent beings. Their identities are parasitic upon social phenomena such as human relationships and values. If this is accepted, then plainly phenomena beyond the individual person will feature in the identity conditions of persons: something which is incompatible with ontological individualism. (*See* especially Taylor (1989) and MacIntyre (1999) for convincing developments of this argument.)

Turning now to ethical individualism. Against this it can be argued that the ideal liberal individual which it generates is in fact an ethically impoverished, selfish individual. In other words, the value of the pursuance of autonomy which is given a privileged place within normative individualism, is open to serious challenge. For example, the charge is commonly made that human relationships involve much more than the exercise of, and mutual respect for, the autonomous decisions of those in such relationships. Aspects of the moral life such as love, pity, and care are plausibly held up to be foundational in morality, not autonomy (*see* Reinders, 2000).

Hence it is possible to launch a two-pronged attack at the two foundations of individualism: its ontology of the person, and its ethical implications concerning how persons should act, the moral values they should subscribe to and prioritise.

Before moving on, it is worth emphasising the frequency with which references to individualism occur in the context of discussions of disability. For example, Morris refers to the 'individualist assumptions' which inform ways of defining disability (Morris, 1991, p.180). Veatch wonders whether it is possible to resolve policy questions in relation to questions of the resources to be made available to disabled people 'without simultaneously reexamining the entire structure of our individualistic, competitive society' (Veatch, 1986, p.150).

As seen in the discussion just undertaken, these individualistic assumptions and the view of disablement and of people with disabilities that they generate all stem from a Cartesian picture of the person, one in which the independence of the individual is stressed. The independence has an ontological sense, as we have seen, but it also has a moral sense. Each of these senses poses a threat to the moral standing of disabled people, and each can be responded to convincingly.

Having shown how Cartesian conceptions of the person influence conceptions of disablement, we can now turn to the second main view of the person mentioned above, physicalism. (For the sake of simplicity I am using 'physicalism' to include *both* substance and property physicalism; in other words it is a thesis in which all substances and all properties are physical ones (*see* Kim, 1995).)

Physicalism

Having spent some time setting out the Cartesian view, and its implications for disablement we turn now to the second main option when considering the nature of the person.

If it is implausible to think of human persons as composed of separable mental and physical substances, should we conceive of them as wholly physical things? This proposal at least does not face the same problems as the Cartesian one, since there is no problem of interaction to account for. It is plain that one physical event can cause another. And it is not ontologically extravagant in the way the dualist theory is.

The main difficulty with this view, though, has been whether it can do justice to the apparently non-physical elements of human life, namely consciousness, the emotions, sensations and beliefs. Is it plausible to regard these apparently mental phenomena as, instead, simply physical events, perhaps in the nervous system?

It should be added that this position, physicalism, also motivates another form of ontological individualism. For according to it the nature of the individual person is determined by the physical make-up of the brain. Those who hold extreme forms of genetic determinism can also be charged with holding a view of the person which is a form of ontological individualism. For in this view too, the nature of the individual person is determined entirely by features internal to it, in this case genetic constitution.

Although the debate concerning physicalist accounts of the person cannot be regarded as conclusively settled one way or the other, it is fair to say that many philosophers have articulated strong arguments to reject such a 'reductionist' position: one in which mental phenomena are nothing more than physical phenomena, are reduced to them. For, they suggest, how can the experiences of, say, appreciating a great work of art, or a spectacular natural scene, or of parenthood simply be a matter of 'neurones firing'? In the view of many, the mental aspects of these phenomena cannot adequately be captured by their physical descriptions, by descriptions of them in physical terms (*see* e.g. McGinn, 1982; Macdonald, 1989).

Pain has been a particular sticking point. For, the argument runs, if anything is central to pain it is the way it feels. This is, of course, experienced by the person enduring the pain in a unique way. No one can experience another's pain in the exact way, through the exact channels, that they experience it. In contrast to this, physical states are of course publicly available, at least in principle. Hence given suitable equipment it would be possible to see the relevant neurones firing which were said to be – to constitute – pain states. The essentially public nature of physical states is then contrasted with the essentially private nature of pain states. The conclusion is that these differ to such an extent that pain simply cannot just be equivalent to a sequence of physical events in the nervous system (*see* e.g. McGinn, 1982; Macdonald, 1989).

Arguments of this kind have led theorists towards the third option mentioned previously, emergentism.

Emergentism

Emergentism anchors mental states in the physical domain in that it allows the dependency of mental states upon physical states. Thus, unlike Cartesian dualism it denies the separability of the mental and physical realms; and unlike Cartesian dualism it does not posit a 'mental substance', only mental properties. Unlike physicalism, emergentism does not claim that mental states are reducible to physical ones. So according to a view of this kind, human beings would typically be physical beings capable of exemplifying mental properties such as consciousness, sensation and thought. Of course, some human beings, dead ones and those in persistent vegetative states (PVS), may not be capable of exemplifying mental properties.

It is fair to say that the emergentist line is generally considered the most plausible of the three theories identified here, though all three have their problems. The reasons for favouring emergentism are as follows. The separation of the mental and physical realms proposed in the dualist approach is hard to accept. It generates severe difficulties in accounting for mental–physical causation. The apparently empirically close relationship between mental and physical phenomena is impossible to account for. And dualism is also ontologically extravagant. The physicalist line avoids the difficulties which beset Cartesian dualism but brings another insuperable problem. This is the problem of reducing mental properties to physical ones. The emergentist view respects the empirically close relations between mental and physical properties. It is not ontologically extravagant. And it does not seek to reduce mental phenomena to physical phenomena (though it acknowledges the dependence of the former on the latter).

It will help, then in what follows if we bear these three positions in mind. And also bear in mind that the third position, emergentism, is the one which is being taken here as the most plausible.

Emergentism and disablement

To see how disabling conditions can be understood within this philosophical view of the person, let us consider quickly a range of disabling conditions and see how they can be understood within the philosophical background of emergentism. Take conditions such as syndrome Z. Here the relevant physical impairment leads to intellectual disability. Given that within the emergentist perspective a certain level of sophistication in physical structures, such as those of the nervous system, leads to the emergence of mental properties, the characteristic signs of syndrome Z would stem from some failure in the organisation of the sufferer's physical structures. Of course this is entirely in keeping with current orthodoxy.

If one were to consider syndrome Z from a dualist position though, it is much more puzzling to explain. For if the physical and mental realms are separable, how can any physical anomaly play any causal role in any mental phenomenon, such as constant pain or intellectual disablement? And from the physicalist perspective, for reasons given above, it would be problematic to characterise the pain accompanying syndrome Z in purely physical terms. So even though much remains vague within the emergentist line, it seems a more adequate philosophical framework to explain conditions such as syndrome Z.

What of sensory disabilities? Once again, the empirically close links between certain physical structures and the presence or absence of certain senses strongly implies the inadequacy of a dualist position. There are no known cases of the sense of sight surviving in the absence of an optic nerve (or some synthetic substitute); nor are there likely to be. It seems most accurate to think of the experience of seeing, and of sensing in general, as something mental. The feelings of pain, the sensations of taste, touch, sight and sound are all mental phenomena. But their presence and their integrity depends upon the presence of certain physical structures, the relevant parts of the nervous system, or perhaps for some kinds of mental phenomena the nervous system as a whole. Although these points don't demonstrate the inadequacy of dualism they make it sound extremely implausible. As for physicalism and sensory disabilities, this again faces difficulties in adequately characterising mental phenomena in physical terms – if we accept that sensory experience is indeed mental, as proposed here.

From an emergentist perspective, sensory disabilities seem less problematic in terms of explaining their occurrence. Given the dependence of mental phenomena upon physical structures, absence of, or malformation of such structures may well be implicated in the absence of relevant mental phenomena, be this sensory experience, or indeed intellectual disability. So the emergentist perspective once again provides at least an intelligible framework within which to try to seek further explanations of the presence or absence of disabling conditions.

With reference to physical disabilities, all three of the philosophical positions could claim to be able to account for these. Within dualism a missing limb, say, could be accounted for within the physical realm, though of course other philosophical problems with the view remain. And physicalism can similarly account for physical disabilities such as a missing limb. No problems arise here for the emergentist line either. Overall, though, from what has been said so far, the emergentist view does appear to be the most adequate.

In making these points about the emergentist position, I do not wish to overstate its adequacy. It still has problems from a philosophical perspective. These include problems concerning mental causation: if the mental is dependent upon the physical, how can mental phenomena have physical effects, e.g. a decision to raise one's hand causes one's hand to move. How is that possible? Also, what exact level of 'complexity' in physical organisation is necessary for the emergence of mental phenomena? Still further, aren't the relations between the mental and physical realms still quite opaque? It is problematic to equate very specific kinds of neurological events with very specific kinds of mental events (such as thoughts about one's work). However, in spite of these problems this approach does seem the least inadequate of the three we have considered here.

There are further points which need to be stressed, in order to resist charges of oversimplification. The emergentist line as described here still maintains a dualism of a sort. The dualism is between physical properties and mental properties (not mental substance, as in Cartesian dualism). It may be pointed out that such a dualism – even though not a substance dualism – is still problematic in its application to disablement. The criticism may be advanced that this division between mental and physical is far too simplistic and neat. For, it may be continued, disabling conditions have both mental and physical aspects, and these interrelate, and even intermingle. Conditions such as multiple sclerosis (MS), for example, have both mental and physical aspects which interrelate. Thus feelings of being physically weak and fatigued, though mental, are shot through with physical symptoms too. Conversely, suppose one morning one is unable to do a task one had hitherto been capable of undertaking without problem, say a short 100 metre walk to buy a newspaper. One's limbs simply won't get one to the shop and back. This may lead one to feel much worse, and again to lead to even greater physical limitations: one may not undertake the short trip again for fear of being unable to complete it without severe discomfort.

On this general topic, it is interesting to consider some remarks of Wendell (1996). She has myalgic encephalomyelitis (ME) and in a discussion of the body in disabling conditions accompanied by chronic pain she speaks of a 'transcendence of the body' (Wendell, 1996, p.165). The proposal is that rather than being 'as one' with her body, she regards it as an 'observer' might:

> I observe what is happening as a phenomenon, attend to it, tolerate the cognitive dissonance that results from, for example, feeling depressed or nauseated when there is nothing obviously depressing or disgusting going on, accommodate to it as best I can, and wait for it to pass (Wendell, 1996, p.174).

Here then Wendell seems to be stating that she can distance herself, cognitively, from some of the symptoms of her condition, can 'monitor' them and cope with them. This 'transcendence' of the body, to use her term, is plainly not a Cartesian transcendence in which the mind can free itself of the body and be pain-free, nausea-free etc. Rather it is a kind of 'psychic distancing'. (*See also* Toombs' references to her attempts to 'separate' herself from her body (Toombs, 1995, p.18); and Murphy's references to his 'Disembodied self' (Murphy, 1987, p.23), and to his 'radical dissociation from the body' (Murphy, 1987, p.86).)

The emergentist approach seems congenial to explication of this kind of mode of dealing with symptoms. For unlike the Cartesian dualist line, it accepts the close relations between bodily and mental phenomena. And unlike the physicalist line it permits some distancing between the mental and physical domains as seems to occur in Wendell's account.

In criticism of her, it can be pointed out that she seems to place sensations of physical pain within the physical domain. On p.170 of her book, she speaks of 'physical pain'. But strictly speaking, all pain is mental even though, of course, it may have a physical cause. It is mental because it is defined by the way it feels, by the way it is experienced.

Wendell's discussion, and the idea of a (non-Cartesian) 'transcendence of the body' raises neatly a distinction sometimes made between the body-as-lived and the 'object-body' (Merleau-Ponty, 1945/1962; Gadow, 1982). Wendell's reflections in the quote above concerning the strategy of transcendence, are plainly made from the perspective of the person 'living in the body', they reflect the perspective of the lived body. The perspective of the object body is that of the observer. Wendell's description of her strategy here shows how important the lived body perspective is in coping with chronic illness. For, viewed from the perspective of the object body, it seems unlikely that such a strategy would occur to one.

It should be stressed that Wendell's strategy of 'transcending the body' does not entail that the person is separable from the body. The lived body is still embodied even if a strategy of the kind devised by Wendell (and others) suggests that 'disembodying' is possible.

Having considered three philosophical views of the person, I want now to turn to a controversial distinction which has been applied to philosophical discussion of the moral standing of humans with serious intellectual disabilities. The distinction claimed is that between persons and human beings.

Persons and human beings

As mentioned early in Part One, recent writers in medical ethics have proposed the idea that a distinction can be drawn between persons and human beings (Tooley, 1972; Harris, 1985; Singer, 1993). The suggestion is that there may be persons who are not humans, and conversely there may be humans who fail to meet the criteria for personhood.

The basis for the distinction is described as follows by Harris: 'a person will be any being capable of valuing its own existence' (Harris, 1985, p.18). This requires some basic level of cognitive sophistication, conceptualisation of past, present and future, and the capacity for self-consciousness; that is, for second-order reflection on one's first-order thoughts and experiences. Harris is explicit that at least some chimpanzees can meet such criteria (Harris, 1985, p.20), and that some humans may not (Harris, 1985, p.25). Neonates, those with very severe intellectual disabilities, and extreme forms of dementia all count as human beings but not as persons by the criterion offered by Harris (and also Singer, 1993, p.87).

It should be emphasised that this is an *ontological* distinction: a distinction between types of existent things. However, it is used to generate a specific claim in the sphere of ethics. This is that the person/human being distinction clearly makes intelligible the idea that some human beings have a lower moral status than others. Those human beings that are persons, if one accepts the distinction, have a higher moral standing than those human beings that are not persons. This is basically because they can be wronged in more ways, notably they can be deprived of a future in a way in which non-persons cannot be so deprived, and therefore harmed (Harris, 1985, p.17).

The idea of moral status or, equivalently, moral standing was explained in Part One ('Why bother ...?'). The point made in explication of the idea was that the moral standing ascribed to a class of beings (worms, farm animals, humans etc) can be determined from the way they are typically acted towards. Think now about the different ways in which foetuses with genetically based disabling traits are acted towards, when compared with the way in which other foetuses are acted towards. We try to eliminate the former group but do not take active steps to eliminate members of the latter group. In addition, in the UK, termination of a foetus with no genetic anomalies is not legal once the foetus is above 24 weeks old. But termination of a foetus in which disabling traits have been detected is legal right up until the moment of birth (*Human Fertilisation and Embryology Act 1990*, section 37; also Morris, 1991, p.67).

Still further, up until relatively recently (the last 20 years) the practice of allowing neonates to die solely on the grounds that they had a disability was not uncommon (*see* Kuhse and Singer, 1985). Thus infants who could have lived were deliberately neglected by healthcare professionals on the grounds that they had disabling traits. Given what was said about moral status, it seems reasonable to conclude that foetuses and neonates with disabling traits were, and perhaps still are, accorded a lower moral standing than non-disabled foetuses and neonates.

Moreover, the practice of screening, diagnosing and terminating on grounds of disability in the foetus may even imply that the moral status of disabled adults is less than that of non-disabled adult human beings. Such a view seems to be expressed in the following quote from a book by Professor John Harris:

> ... anyone who thinks that the detection of handicap in the foetus is a good reason for abortion, must accept that such an individual is, or will become, less valuable than one without such handicap, less valuable because less worth saving or less entitled to life (Harris, 1985, p.7).

In addition, of course, the promulgation of the person/human being distinction might reasonably be judged to impugn the moral standing of intellectually disabled people. For the person/human being distinction is made on grounds that centre on cognitive capacity. And anyone judged to be intellectually disabled is being defined by their cognitive incapacity, thus, it may be felt, impugning their moral standing when compared to humans who do not have serious (or even mild) cognitive incapacities.

So the criteria for personhood adhered to by a number of influential contemporary philosophers seem to jeopardise the moral standing of intellectually disabled people. And the passage from Harris quoted earlier suggests that this can be generalised to extend to people with any disability that is currently screened for prenatally. Thus acceptance of the person/human being distinction – tacit or explicit – may be one reason for screening and termination on grounds of disability in the foetus (specifically intellectual disability).

To summarise: widely prevalent conceptions of what it is to be a person generate the presumption that disability is a bad thing. For, according to such conceptions of the person, the presence of disability in a person is considered to impugn something of great significance. This is either the moral standing of that individual, relative to other human beings, or, in the case of individualism, the view that disability fatally compromises the status of the disabled person as a philosophically legitimate person.

As mentioned, strictly speaking, the person/human being distinction is one within the sphere of ontology, and can be understood without reference to moral concerns. But again as noted, it has been exploited for these purposes. As may be expected, the distinction and the use made of it by ethicists such as Harris and Singer is extremely controversial, especially amongst disabled people (Johnson, 2003; and the 'Not Dead Yet' organisation www.notdeadyet.org). But one can see the appeal of the distinction. If it is applied to humans in PVS, say, it does seem that a human person has more to lose, and has more interests than a human in PVS. So given that, it seems reasonable to claim that it is a greater wrong to end the life of a person than a human in PVS. I will refrain from comment on other disabling conditions, but as indicated it does seem plausible to me that the distinction generates a credible position in morality at least when considering the plight of humans in PVS. To allow this, of course, is not to allow that all disabled human beings have a lower moral standing than 'able' human beings. Our deliberations in Part Two strongly made the case against this in showing that disabled individuals have the capacity to lead a good human life. It follows that the moral standing which should be accorded to them is full, not partial.

Disablement and personal identity

The points we have been discussing thus far in Part Three have concerned general ontological positions applied to persons/human beings. The position proposed as most plausible is that of emergentism. We have not yet touched upon the topic of identity. The question to be posed is 'is disability ever an identity-constituting characteristic (property) of a human being?'. The claim that disability can be such an identity-constituting characteristic will be called 'the identity claim'. (The quote from Oliver at the start of this part shows that, for him, disability is such an identity-constituting characteristic (Oliver, 1990, p.xiii). Thus he endorses the 'identity claim'.)

It should be said that whole notion of identity when applied to questions regarding the identity of persons has been horrendously problematic (*see* e.g. Williams, 1973; Shoemaker and Swinburne, 1984; Parfit, 1986; Baker, 2000 and numerous other contributions). However, in the main we make judgements to the effect that 'A is the same person now as he was last week', all the time in our day-to-day dealings with one another, providing a philosophically adequate account of personal identity has proved very difficult.

It is important to note that the issue at stake is not simply about a person undergoing changes. Of course it seems most plausible to suppose one person undergoes many changes throughout a lifetime. Yet, from a commonsense perspective at least, there is something in virtue of which they remain the same person throughout these changes. The problem of personal identity is the problem of specifying just what this 'something in virtue of which' is.

Discussions of personal identity within mainstream English-speaking philosophy have tried to pursue two main options, one which focuses on the body, and the other which focuses on psychological characteristics.

Theories of personal identity have generally appealed either to physical or psychological continuity (*see* e.g. Nozick, 1981, Chapter 1). Physical continuity theories focus on the brain of the person and tend to lapse into 'brain possession' theories in which personal identity follows the brain. Hence, in swapping the brains of prime ministers, Thatcher and Blair identity would follow brain possession. In psychological continuity theories, what matters most is psychological continuity and, at least theoretically, it is held that such continuity can survive the detaching of the relevant set of psychological properties from the body of the subject (*see* Dennett, 1981). For example, if a 'thought extraction device' could transfer my psychological properties – my memories etc. – onto a computer program, according to psychological continuity accounts, 'I' would survive (again, *see* Dennett, 1981).

It is fair to say that both kinds of theories are generally deemed to be unsuccessful. Those that focus on the body, it is objected, cannot do justice to the place of psychological characteristics in identity. To see this, suppose Blair's brain is subjected to the 'thought extraction device' invented by Shoemaker and Swinburne (1984), and that Thatcher's psychological traits (her memories, cognitive habits etc.) are 'inserted' into Blair's brain. Proponents of the physical continuity view have to claim the resulting person is still Blair. Psychological continuity theorists are forced to conclude the resulting person is Thatcher.

Others find neither of these conclusions satisfactory. They query the crudity of the method involved and the omission to consider how such a swap could work in practice (Wilkes, 1993). How could Thatcher's 'cognitive habits' plug into Blair's body?

A further option has focused on the *origin* of individuals. In a discussion of the effects of gene therapy upon identity, Persson (1995) has argued for an 'origination theory' in which: 'the numerical identity of a human person is entirely determined by the identity of the (foetal) body in which he originates' (Persson, 1995, p.22). Thus according to him identity is fixed by origin.

However, against Persson, and others attracted to 'origination theses' of identity, it should be noted that philosophers tempted by an appeal to origin have differing views on precisely when this is. For Persson it is the foetal stage of development (*see* Persson, 1995, p.22); for Kripke it is the zygote (Kripke, 1981, p.113); and for Harris it is the gametes (Harris, 1998, p.80) (i.e. *that* sperm, and *that* ovum). These differences indicate a problem in the appeal to origin: namely, when to stop searching for it.

This is in fact a serious problem for origination theses. To see this, consider that the disagreement between Harris and Kripke, presumably, stems from differing opinions about what actually determines the nature of the individual person. For Kripke it is the fertilised egg, for Harris it is the individual gametes. They arrive at differing views on origin because they apply the following principle in the same way but arrive at differing answers. The principle is: the relevant considerations in origin are those that affect the properties of the individual whose identity is in question. But of course the genetic constitution of the producer of the gametes (sperm, ovum) is relevant too, as is the producer of the sperm and ovum which led to the existence of the contributors of sperm and ovum, and so on. In short, origination theses lead to an infinite regress in the search for origin.

Further, a paper by Belshaw (2000) calls seriously into question the Kripkean version of the origination thesis; his objection applies also to the theses of Harris and Persson. In summary, Belshaw invites us to consider just why the sperm and egg are considered important in identity questions. Among the reasons why they are so considered is the view that they have an impact on the psychological traits of the resulting child. Thus, focus just on sperm. This is presumably considered important because of its influence on characteristics such as the psychological characteristics, intelligence etc. of the resulting child. A different sperm from a different father may result in differences in these. But, Belshaw continues, suppose that sperm is 'informationally neutral' (Belshaw, 2000, p.269), and hence it makes no contribution to the psychology of the child. Then, it is argued, the Kripkean line faces two difficulties. First, in the hypothetical situation where sperm is informationally neutral, the Kripkean line claims, implausibly, that something which 'makes no difference to the obvious and surface characteristics of a thing, does matter' (Belshaw, 2000, p.269). And second, that characteristics which do matter to identity judgements, such as 'surface' psychological characteristics, do not matter. Again, this is implausible. I am sympathetic to these objections.

Anyway these and other concerns with tradtional approaches to the problem of personal identity led one eminent philosopher to propose an extremely radical position.

Famously, Parfit's conclusion is that identity is not what matters (Parfit, 1984, p.255). Rather, what matters is that a person exhibiting a degree of psychological continuity with oneself survives into the future. Thus, a person that is psychologically continuous with you can reside in the body of another person, e.g. one with whom one has had a close relationship. On this view, then, persons do not 'map' 1:1 with bodies but can be spread across numerous bodies. Importantly, the continued existence of a person – their survival – differs from the way survival is understood in a lay sense of survival. In the lay view, survival is not a matter of degree, but is an 'all or nothing' matter. Put differently, in the approach to the problem advanced by Parfit, survival is a *qualitative* relation only. However, some telling objections have been levelled at such a position.

Schectman (1996) argues that survival in the lay sense certainly does matter in questions of personal identity. She does this by identifying four features of our 'prephilosophical' (1996, p.13) thought about personal identity. These are 'survival, moral responsibility, self-interested concern, and compensation' (Schectman, 1996, p.2). She suggests that psychological continuity is important precisely because of its connections to identity: she claims 'the four features require numerical identity' (Schectman, 1996, p.52).

In order to try to make this claim stick, Schectman reminds us that psychological continuity as conceived within psychological continuity theories such as Parfit's, is a qualitative relation. Hence, successive stages of selves are more or less psychologically continuous; continuity is not an all or nothing matter, it is a matter of degree only. This is contrasted with the notion of numerical identity in which identity is not a matter of degree: two things either are or are not identical. And, as noted, she claims that the importance of the four features requires numerical, not mere qualitative, identity.

For example, consider 'self-interested concern' (Schectman, 1996, p.52). Of this she writes:

> Self-interested concern is an emotion that is appropriately felt only toward my own self and not toward someone like me. We all know the difference between fearing for our own pain and fearing for the pain of someone else (Schectman, 1996, p.52).

She goes on to point out we might care more about the pain which another person may have to endure – e.g. if it is one's child. But the important difference is not the degree of fear felt, but the crucial difference between fearing pain one is oneself about to endure, and fearing pain another person is about to endure.

In relation to another of the four features, compensation, she writes, 'only benefits to me can compensate me for present sacrifices' (Schectman, 1996, p.52). So my working hard can be explained by my anticipating a lengthy holiday by way of a reward. But how could such actions be explained if the rewards were to go to another person? Hence, Schectman's claim is that the language of compensation requires that of numerical identity: that it is me and not someone else who is compensated for my hard work. She makes the same point with respect to moral responsibility (Schectman, 1996, p.53).

With regard to survival, Schectman writes,

> qualitative similarity does not seem enough for survival – the existence of a person in the future who has beliefs, values, desires and so on very like mine does not seem to guarantee my survival any more than the existence of someone with a psychological life very different from mine does (Schectman, 1996, p.53).

She elaborates this by suggesting that she,

> would rather wake up tomorrow with partial amnesia than be smothered in my sleep by the evil genius who has also brainwashed my next-door neighbour to exhibit my psychological make-up (ibid).

So this attack, mounted by Schectman, is an attempt to take on a celebrated account of personal identity and to try to show it to be unsuccessful. The attack demonstrates that acceptance of the Parfitian solution would generate such a radical overhaul of our conception of agency and moral agency that it is unlikely to be true.

Other commentators have made similar attempts (e.g. Ricoeur, 1992), again largely prompted by the view that our personal identity judgements are generally successful, yet an account of the philosophical grounds of personal identity seems elusive within the constraints of the English-speaking analytic philosophical tradition.

No doubt the dissatisfaction with standard approaches within the analytic tradition led at least some philosophers to consider other approaches and to be suspicious of the constraints within which theorising on the subject of personal identity standardly takes place (*see* e.g. Ricoeur, 1992; Schectman, 1996). One such key constraint is what can be called the 'essential properties constraint'.

The essential properties constraint

It may be objected that there is no prospect of success for the identity claim due to the fact that disability is a contingent property of persons. Or, alternatively, it may be claimed that disability can be identity constituting but only if it is genetic in origin.

Both these responses share methodological commitment to what we can call the essential properties constraint (EPC). This is the constraint that questions of personal identity turn upon the possession or loss of a set of properties deemed essential. Thus in the response which claims disability is contingent, it is supposed that disabling characteristics do not fall within the class of essential properties. In a response which allowed that disabling characteristics are identity constituting, it would be due to their falling within the class of essential properties; as mentioned, the most likely candidates for such a class would be genetic characteristics.

So if one subscribes to EPC it is very unlikely that one will take disabilities to be identity constituting. This certainly holds true of people such as Jenny Morris for she became disabled as a result of an accident and so her disability has no genetic component. I suppose one might hold that MS has a genetic origin and so claim that Toombs' disability is identity constituting. But I want to discount that possibility here and consider the more radical proposal that EPC can be jettisoned in accounts of personal identity.

Why jettison essential properties contraint?

First, of course, it is problematic to find any identity-constituting features of a person, especially at the intentional level. For any such feature, it seems, is such that a person might not have exemplified it.

Thus we think of Florence Nightingale as a nurse yet, had her life turned out differently, she might never have gone into nursing. We think of Margaret Thatcher as a former prime minister but she might never have gone into politics.

Secondly, it seems, any physical characteristics that we actually do happen to possess we might not have. Nowadays it is possible to change a person's gender, and in future it may be possible to replace human body parts with bionic substitutes.

Thus it seems that all the properties one actually does exemplify are contingent. They are characteristics which one might not have acquired and, therefore by accounts of identity constrained by EPC they cannot define one's identity.

Certainly, those properties which characterise us, namely our appearance, self-conception, self-project, and narrative are surely contingent. (See below for exposition of these ideas.)

Third, as MacIntyre has indicated (1981, p.217) the idea of 'strict' identity exploited in the EPC is itself inseparable from a less strict understanding of identity – one which is relied upon in our ordinary identity judgements regarding persons.

It is the apparent contingency of properties of persons which has generated such problems for attempts to develop a robust theory of personal identity in philosophy. Psychological continuity ignores the importance of the physical aspects of our being. Physical continuity theories ignore the psychological aspects of our being. 'Closest continuer' theories are vulnerable to the objection that what matters to one is that one survives, not that one's 'closest continuer' does (Baker, 2000, p.127). Origination theses are vulnerable in the way described above. Jettisoning numerical identity as favoured by Parfit seems simply too radical to be plausible. In the light of this, I want to suggest an alternative approach, one which jettisons the EPC, and which, as will be seen, is highly congenial to the view of disablement as identity constituting.

Narrative identity and disablement

The previous discussion of theories of personal identity and of EPC strongly suggests that accounts of personal identity that seek to respect EPC are doomed to failure. Such attempts motivate the extreme of denying that identity matters (viz Parfit, 1984). But as we saw, this is simply not a credible option. One explanation for the failure of theories of personal identity of the kind discussed so far is that two differing concepts of identity are implicated in identity judgements. One is a sense of identity which accords great weight to character, moral agency and other apparently contingent psychologically grounded aspects. The other concept is one which applies unproblematically to inanimate objects, which serves to anchor their numerical identity over time. But, the explanation runs, the former concept is 'constitutionally incapable' (Schectman, 1996, p.7) of being captured by the latter. (This analysis is also presented by Ricoeur, 1991.)

Of course this explanation of the failure falls short of providing a solution to it. But, borrowing from Ricoeur and others, I attempt to sketch a theory of personal identity below. As will be seen, it is one congenial to the proposal that disablement can be identity-constituting. The theory follows Ricoeur in maintaining that a theory of personal identity should provide the resources capable of answering the question 'who?' for the person whose identity is in question. Also, the theory exploits the idea of narrativity especially as presented by MacIntyre (1981).

To take the first of these ideas, what Ricoeur is getting at is this. Suppose one poses the question to another person 'who are you?'. There is a clear sense in which simply giving one's name in response fails to answer the question. Suppose the person answers by providing only their name or their national insurance number. Unless one already knows some additional facts about the person, these answers are at best partial. The 'additional facts' must encompass some details of the life of the person concerned, such as where they live, whether or not they have children, whether or not they are working, what their interests are and so on. A legitimate answer to the question 'who are you?', it is being contended here, must include or presuppose awareness of the kinds of features of the person's life just described. It is reasonable to claim that in providing these further facts one is providing extracts from the person's life story or (equivalently) their narrative.

This now takes us on to MacIntyre's narrative conception of the person, which he summarises thus:

> [It is the] concept of a self whose unity resides in the unity of a narrative which links birth to life to death as narrative beginning to middle to end (MacIntyre, 1981, p.205).

In other words, the life of a person will have a beginning, a middle and an end – just as a narrative will be so structured. The narrative of a person will have a certain 'unity' about it, which contributes to its being the narrative of one person and not another, again just as a story has a unity which makes it one story and not another. Such narratives provide the resources to answer the question 'who?' since they specify a life story, or part of one.

Certain features of a narrative contribute to the unity noted by MacIntyre. The first is temporality. Inevitably, the narrative of a person will have a temporal structure to it, stretching across past, present and future. Human experience itself too is temporal in character: persons have a past, live in a present, and are oriented towards a future.

It is evident that temporality, although a necessary feature of a narrative, will not be sufficient to characterise a person's narrative. The reason is that relations within narratives, in addition to being temporal relations, are relations of intelligibility. Stories don't simply run across periods of time, their integrity – 'unity' – derives from connections of intelligibility between events occurring at one period of time and events occurring at other periods of time.

It is worth adding that human agency is itself narratival. Human actions can be explained in narrative terms. Take the trivial act of a person leaving the room to buy a newspaper. The act must be presented in the form of a story, with a beginning, middle and end.

The intelligibility and unity of a narrative is also dependent upon values. To see this, consider Taylor's (1989) proposal that the kind of trivial mini-narrative just described nests within the larger narrative of a person concerning the values and aims of the person. Thus, for example, the person's desire to purchase a newspaper may derive from a broader aim, to keep abreast of current affairs. And this aim in turn may nest within a still broader conception of what a good person is, say, one in which such a person is well-informed about contemporary political affairs. (*See also* MacIntyre, 1981, pp.209–10 for this kind of analysis.)

So here it is seen that an act motivated by one value, the purchase of a newspaper, nests within a broader value-orientation, specifically one concerning the kind of person one aspires to be (in this example, one who is politically well informed).

In further explication of the role that values play in the narrative account of the person, consider Taylor's suggestion that all persons are living an answer to the question 'how should I live?'. One's own answer to this seems manifested by the way one actually acts. (Again, *see also* MacIntyre, 1981, pp.218–19.)

Hence the claim can be advanced that the person, in its very nature is narratival. The narrative is structured by relations of temporality and intelligibility. Actions are narratival in constitution and their intelligibility derives from further aspects of the narrative of the person. These aspects include the person's aspirations and values. Over the course of a life, a life story captures the life of a person. This life story manifests the identity of the person and provides an answer to the question 'who?'.

This example helps to show how personal identity relates to a self-conception, a view of the kind of person one aspires to be. It is in this way that one's acts manifest an answer to the question 'how should I live?', for answering this presupposes some conception of the kind of person one sees oneself as, or aspires to be.

Thus the identities of persons inescapably involve moral values. And this is something we will return to later when considering the five structuring concepts of personal existence.

Since descriptions of actions that figure in a narrative are inevitably open to re-interpretation, a narrative will never be definitively closed. Thus, an act described at one time as one of generosity may later be redescribed as one of manipulation as events unfold further. For example, suppose Robert Maxwell's shady business dealings had not been uncovered until some years after his death. Prior to the exposure of such facts, his narrative may well have been that of a philanthropist, yet subsequently be revised to that of an untrustworthy businessman.

A further noteworthy feature of this narrative account of the person is that personal identity will require the resources of a natural language. This is because it is only possible to formulate a 'self-conception', given the resources of a natural language. So this idea of the person is not individualistic in the way in which other views are, in particular the Cartesian view. For the very idea of the person requires the existence of social phenomena, notably a language, and, as we have also seen, a set of moral parameters within which persons judge which kinds of lives they wish to lead, or, more strikingly, in which they live their answers to the question 'how should I live?'.

With reference to role of the human body in all this, Kerby suggests that bodies serve as 'sites of narration' (Kerby, 1991, p.4). Hence some kind of anchor is provided for the ascriptions of personal identity.

Hence, stories said to constitute the identities of persons will include references to events that are not themselves language independent, and that are permanently revisable.

In a nutshell, then, the account of narrative identity provided so far suggests that personal identity is given by a narrative, a life story. This is anchored at one level in a person's physical nature, the fact they are inevitably embodied, and at another level in psychological characteristics. These include the kind of 'sedimentations' of character referred to above, in the form of commitments to certain value orientations. It is these which render explicable a person's actions in relation to the events of which she is a part. It is sequences of such events that are described in a narrative.

Also, four key aspects of narratives have been identified: their temporal form (beginnings, middles, ends etc.); the fact that relations between the stages of a narrative are relations of intelligibility; the inescapable value component of narrative; and their inescapably social nature. Now, in applying this to 'the identity claim', it will be necessary to specify what we will describe as 'five essential structuring concepts of personal existence'.

Five essential structuring concepts of personal existence

As noted, narratives must be temporal, and the stages must be related by relations of intelligibility. What I would like to set out now are five 'structuring concepts' which provide the *form* of narratives. The narrative of a person will inevitably include each of the five structuring concepts to be introduced now. Each concept represents an essential aspect of personal existence, and each concept will be 'completed' during the life of the individual. Personal identity will be given by the mode in which each concept is completed. This will differ for individual persons (not least because two persons cannot occupy identical spatio-temporal trajectories). Within each of the five concepts, constituting properties will feature, though no single concept will have resources capable of giving personal identity, of answering the question 'who?'. In other words, answering the question 'who?' will involve more than specifying the content of any single structuring concept. To see this, note that specifying the spatio-temporal trajectory of a person will not answer the question 'who?' for that person because it will contain nothing about that person's values, or life plans.

The descriptions provided within each of the five concepts will provide the content of the narrative. The form of the narrative will be provided by the five structuring concepts.

Consider, then, five essential aspects of personal existence:

(1) persons exist in space
(2) they also exist in time
(3) persons are embodied: they stand in a relationship to a body
(4) persons have a self-conception (a conception of the kind of person they are aspiring to be)
(5) persons are engaged in the pursuit of a self-project which will realise their self-conception.

I take it that aspects 1 and 2 are uncontroversial, in particular, given the earlier endorsement of emergentism. Human beings live in time, and, because they necessarily have a physical component to their existence, they exist in space too.

To add a little more, consider space. Just as it is clear that the narratives of persons are temporally structured, so too are they spatially structured: all our actions take place in space, persons are spatially located, and stand in spatial relations to objects, places and other persons.

It is easy to show how central such relations are in the narratives of persons. For example, reference to one's place of birth or upbringing is a likely component of a narrative; obviously such places are spatially located. Similarly, the distance one is from loved ones, places one would like to visit, places one has to visit (school, church, work) each characteristically figure in one's narrative. Also, at the everyday level, the natures of the actions that persons under-take are partially determined by spatial relations. One may rise in time to take children to school. The time this takes depends, of course, upon the distance between the school and where one lives. Similarly, in planning the rest of the day's activities, it is necessary to take into account the spatial relations between one's various destinations.

Also, it is possible to distinguish objective spatial relations from spatial relations as they are lived, as they are perceived by the person. For example, when one is a small child, the distance from the kitchen to the lounge may seem vast compared to the distance it seems when one is an adult. The conception one has of sizes also differs. To the child, an adult seems enormous, but this changes when one grows up; examples can be multiplied indefinitely. The point is that a distinction can be made between spatial relations as these seem to the perceiving subject, and as they objectively are. This contrast may be signalled by the distinction between subjective (spatial relations as they are lived, experienced, by the person) and objective space.

Consider time: this is generally appealed to in philosophical literature as a concept central to, or presupposed by, the concept of the person (e.g. Kant, 1781/1929). On the face of it this seems a reasonable claim. However persons are conceived of, it seems they must be conceived of as located within time. Even the extreme Cartesian view of the person according to which the self is only certain of its existence whilst it is doubting it exists, presupposes a time at which that doubt takes place. And, in less sceptical frames of mind, it is evident that the nature of the existence of persons is essentially temporal. All our thoughts, actions, and emotions have a temporal dimension in the trivial sense in which there is a time at which, or during which, they occur. But further, it is clear that persons are temporal in a deeper sense (Taylor, 1989, p.49). A person has a history, replete with memories, plans for the future. And of course, the present, the time at which one is recollecting the past, envisaging or planning the future, is inescapable for the person. Further, the present is partially determined by the past. The explanation of why one is situated in one place rather than another (say London rather than Aberdeen) necessarily involves reference to past events.

As with the spatial aspect of personal existence, a distinction can be made between objective time and subjective time (Husserl, 1913/ 1962, p.215). As might be expected, this is the distinction between the amount of time a person thinks has elapsed, and the amount of time which has actually elapsed. This distinction points to the possibility of differences in perception of the degree of time which has elapsed during a particular event. Examinees may report that an hour passed by extremely quickly, and seemed more like half an hour. To the invigilator, by contrast, the hour may have felt like two hours. Yet, it is legitimate to claim that, in fact, only one hour passed. Bauby, a person paralysed with locked-in syndrome wrote of his time in hospital, 'Time, motionless in here, gallops out there' (Bauby, 1997, p.108).

The third of our five concepts, embodiment, is complicated partly because of the ambiguity of the term 'embodied'. In one way this can be interpreted in a Cartesian sense such that the person 'occupies' the body, and uses it, so to speak. In this view, the body is a mere instrument of the person. The second interpretation of 'embodied' is an explicit rejection of the Cartesian line implied in the previous interpretation. On this second interpretation, one *is* one's body. Thus it makes no sense to say of a person that they *use* their body as an instrument, for user and used are identical.

This is a complex issue, and observations can be recruited in support of either interpretation. In support of the 'body as instrument' interpretation, Toombs has proposed that her body is an 'obstacle to the self' and that she fears being 'imprisoned by [her] body' (Toombs, 1995, p.11; *see also* Wendell, 1996).

It has become common in recent years to claim that 'one is one's body'. In other words that there is, in fact, no distinction between the person and the body. The view is attributed to Merleau-Ponty (e.g. by Benner, 2000, p.6) and endorsed by others, e.g. Toombs. Yet, in the context of disablement a self/body distinction is often claimed.

Thus Toombs observes that disabled people 'necessarily come to view the world through the medium of their damaged bodies' (Toombs, 1995, p.14). And she refers to a 'changed relationship with one's body' (Toombs, 1995, p.12). Cassell claims that persons with chronic illness are 'in conflict' with their body; that the body is 'untrustworthy' (e.g. one may become incontinent), and that the body is a source of 'humiliation'. He also speaks of a battle in which the person is pitted against the body (Cassell, 1990, pp.56–8; *see also* Gadow, 1982; Bauby, 1997).

One way to characterise these two positions is to refer to them as expressing two models of 'embodiment', what we might term (a) a housing model, and (b) an identity model. (Thus Toombs writes, 'I do not "have" or "possess" a body, I *am* my body' (Toombs, 1993, p.51). In the 'housing model', there is a presumed separability between person and body such that the body imprisons the person. So here the person is embodied but 'embodied' means something like 'entombed', 'housed' or 'encased'.

On such a view there is no question of an identity between that which is 'embodied' and that which is responsible for the 'entombing' so to speak: i.e. no identity between the person and its 'tomb', 'house', or 'case'.

But in the 'identity model', embodiment tends to be employed (following Merleau-Ponty, 1945/1962) to suggest an identity between the person and the body. Recall Toombs again '... I am my body, in that I am an embodied subject' (Toombs, 1993, p.52). In this second model the person *is* the body. In this second use of the idea of embodiment there is an identity between person and body. Hence the idea of the person being distinct from the body, as an obstacle to the person, say, is not coherent. It could only be said that the self is an obstacle to itself. Or, paraphrasing Toombs, the self 'views the world through the medium of itself'.

The coherence of a distinction between self and body may also be elucidated by appeal to the distinction between lived and object body. If we look at the 'I am my body' claim again in the light of this distinction we can say that at the level of the lived body we are indeed embodied persons in the second of the senses identified above. That is the person is identical to the lived body. So, contrary to the remarks of Toombs and Cassell which propose a person/body distinction, if this is understood as the claim 'I am my lived body', then there is in fact no person/body distinction. And the claim that 'I am my body' can be salvaged: the claimed self/body distinction is false when 'body' is understood as 'lived body'.

Thus, the embodiment aspect of human existence needs to be understood as follows. Since embodiment, having a body, is inescapable, humans are embodied. So persons are their bodies. The body can, though, be viewed from two perspectives, as an object, and from the perspective of the lived body. Only the person identical to that body has the latter perspective available to them. Lastly, since persons are their bodies, and since persons are thinking, conscious beings, not machines, the body is properly regarded as a subject, not as an object.

The remark from Kerby earlier, and the account of narrative identity given earlier make it plain that a body will be necessary for the attribution of narrative identity, after all a human being needs a body to be capable of action. And it is reasonable to suppose the identification and re-identification of the person by others depends upon embodiment. In that sense the body provides a 'route' to the person, so to speak. Also, it is likely that bodily aspects will figure in the narrative of persons for reasons to be given shortly.

The fourth and fifth aspects of personal existence are self-conception, and self-project respectively.

In explanation of the idea of a self-conception, begin by considering fairly trivial human actions, such as making a cup of tea. As observed earlier, such acts will take narrative form, having beginnings, middles and ends. But why is the person making the tea? Perhaps they are thirsty, or cold. The actions of persons are intelligible against a wider background or context.

A series of actions such as the taking of exams is made sense of by a person's intention to obtain qualifications. Why do they want to obtain them? Well, to increase the range of employment opportunities open to them, or simply to increase their knowledge of a range of subjects of interest to them.

Here we see again that 'smaller' goals are nested within larger ones. The goal to make tea is nested within the goal of slaking thirst, and ultimately of taking in liquid to stay alive. The goal of passing an exam is again nested within larger goals, e.g. for academic advancement, increase in life opportunities etc.

It is plausible to propose that pursuance, by a person, of broader goals can be understood against a very broad conception of the *kind* of person one wants to be, or of the kind of person one sees oneself as. This very broad conception is what is being termed here a 'self-conception'. Evidently, a self-conception represents a particular value-orientation, since in opting for one rather than another, one is expressing commitment to the view that one kind life is 'better than' another. 'Better than' here returns us again to the discussion of the good human life. For in judging one kind of life as better than another one makes manifest a judgement about the kind of life which one would regard as a good life. (As mentioned, this view of the person is one inspired by the work of Charles Taylor (*see* Taylor, 1989); *see* also van Hooft (1995) from whom I borrow the expression 'self-project').

Turning now to the final aspect of personal existence, that of a self-project. In a nutshell, this can be glossed as the pursuit of a self-conception. A self-project is one's quest to realise one's self-conception. So a description of a self-project will be a description of the strategies a person takes to try to become the kind of person they aspire to be. Thus, a 'mini-narrative' such as a description of a trip to the cinema with one's children should, ultimately, be made intelligible in terms of the person's self-conception. In this example, their self-conception may involve being a good parent and they may view the trip as fostering or cultivating that goal.

As a further illustration of the relationship between a self-conception and a self-project, the footballer David Beckham has a self-conception, an overarching goal: to be a great footballer. His self-project is to become one. His day-to-day acts, mini-narratives, are oriented towards fulfilment of his self-conception.

The narrative of a person includes a description of the attempt to enact a self-project, where this is fuelled by a self-conception.

Overall, then, it is being proposed here that these five aspects of personal existence are bound to feature in the narrative of a person and will manifest the identity of that person. Each aspect corresponds to a structuring concept in a narrative. So the narrative of a person will be structured in terms of these five concepts. Each of the five will be 'completed' during the course of a lifetime. Some aspects of the narrative may even persist after death, as seen in the case of Robert Maxwell. But death is signalled by the cessation of the embodiment component of a narrative, since at death this bodily dimension ceases (the body ceases to function). The narrative may continue, but will then be the narrative of a dead person, not a living one, due to the necessity of the embodiment aspect of human existence.

We have seen how time and space are inescapable features of a narrative since all actions take place in those dimensions. We have seen also that the body of a person will have a central role. Bodies will be central to the narratives of persons in general because they are necessary conditions for acting. And of course bodies are acted upon by others. Bodily presence prompts events which will figure in a narrative. A body will, thus, be necessary for the acquisition and attribution of narrative identity. As noted, it is reasonable to suppose the identification and re-identification of a person by others depends upon embodiment. In that sense the body plays the role of a 'route' to the person.

Bodily aspects will feature in the narratives of persons, partly because of the dimensions of human experience given earlier of which one is embodiment, but also because one's physical appearance, gait, posture and so on are part of what it is to be one. It is on the basis of these aspects of one that others respond to one and therefore physical appearance will have a place in one's narrative at least implicitly.

With reference to particular persons, again it seems plain that one's body is likely to be fundamental to one's narrative. For example, friends recognise each other by their characteristic appearance – their familiar posture, gait, style of clothing and so on. Evidently, countless interactions between persons derive from bodily appearance. Also, it is common to point out that one's bodily appearance often reveals emotions such as anger or apprehension. And it is plausible to suppose that these appearances have a structuring role in the narrative of a person, due to their influence on the character of human interactions. For example, in conversations between persons, if one of the participants appears angry, this is likely to affect the nature of the conversation. Also, of course, one's physical history, in standard cases, is also unique to one. Persons follow a unique spatial trajectory through space and time during their lives.

So both the general claim that embodiment will feature in the narratives of persons, and the specific claim about the role of embodiment in particular narratives seem convincing.

And we have seen how those aspects of personal existence termed 'self-conception' and 'self-project' similarly are central to a narrative. Indeed it is these aspects of a narrative that identify it as that of a person as opposed to that of an inanimate object (since of course one can narrate the creation, existence and destruction of these too in terms of beginnings, middles and ends).

Having set out this general approach to specifying the identities of persons, we return now specifically to its application to disablement.

Disablement and the five structuring concepts

In her book *Pride Against Prejudice* Jenny Morris describes how, at the age of 33, she became disabled. Having hitherto been able-bodied she fell off a wall and injured herself so badly that she lost the use of her legs, permanently. Early on in her study she reports that in the 10 years that elapsed between her becoming disabled and writing the book, she has 'developed an identity as a disabled woman' (Morris, 1991, p.1). She also recounts the way in which other people responded to her. Some were positive, but others found it very difficult to speak to her on an equal basis, so to speak, person to person. She suggests that some people she encountered following her accident indicated they felt her life no longer worth living (Morris, 1991, p.2).

As we have heard, SK Toombs is a person with MS who also advances claims concerning the extent to which this condition, a chronic illness, has affected her life. Like Morris, she too advances claims regarding the relationship between her condition and her identity. Recall her claim that MS poses 'a threat to the self' (Toombs, 1995, p.12). As with Morris, she is conscious of the way in which other people respond to her, for example by addressing her in a condescending manner.

In addition, it is well known that many members of the deaf community regard their deafness as identity-constituting, as part of what it is to be them (*see* e.g. Sacks, 1989; Rée, 1999; and 'A world of their own' by I Mundy, *Washington Post*, 27 March 2002 regarding couples who hope their children will be deaf as they themselves are).

How should these various claims be understood? From a traditional approach to the problem of personal identity, disabling traits are contingent and therefore cannot be identity constituting. As we have heard, traditional approaches are constrained by the essential properties constraint, but the theory just outlined is not so constrained. So it will be important to see how it would apply in either of the kinds of cases just mentioned.

We observed that there are five essential aspects of personal existence:

(1) persons exist in space
(2) they also exist in time
(3) they are embodied
(4) they have a self-conception (a conception of the kind of person one is aspiring to be)
(5) they are engaged in the pursuit of a self-project which will realise their self-conception.

With reference to space, as it is lived (as it is experienced by the person), Toombs (1995) describes how, as her illness has progressed, distances that hitherto had seemed short now seem far away. Getting from one room to another can be exhausting and this makes it seem as though a great distance is being traversed. Also, she describes how even the same 'objective' distance can seem different depending upon the time of day. A journey from her office to a nearby lecture room may be reached without too much effort on the outward journey, but be exhausting when it comes to the return journey.

Given these last points it is easy to show how disablement can impact upon spatial relations as they are experienced by the person. Recall Toombs' example concerning the distance between her office and the classroom. As she writes:

> Loss of mobility ... transforms the character of surrounding space ... what was formerly regarded as 'near' is now experienced as 'far' (Toombs, 1995, p.13).

Hence the distance previously considered near, becomes far. Moreover, even the same distance, considered objectively, can seem distinct when subjectively experienced depending upon one's physical state. Toombs describes how the return journey to her office from the classroom is experienced as being longer than the outward journey, due to the effort expended in teaching.

In addition to how she feels, perceptions of distance are affected by other factors too. She writes,

> The answer to the question 'is it too far?' no longer bears any relation to objective measurement of distance. It depends, rather, on what is between 'here' and 'there'. Are there obstacles that prevent the use of my scooter? Is the terrain suitable for a wheelchair? (Toombs, 1995, p.13).

The extent to which conceptions of space, considered from the perspective of the person, are determined by disablement (and ability) is evident from this quote, and others given above. In effect, objective spatial relations provide little information as to the nature of subjective spatial relations.

A similar story applies in relation to time as it is lived by the person. Tasks which took hardly any time – tying shoelaces, brushing one's teeth, putting on a shirt, now take much longer.

In the description of the mobility problems stemming from her development of MS, Toombs describes the temporal effects of the condition. She describes how moving from her office to the classroom in order to teach changed from being a short distance, occasioning no prior consideration on her part, to a relatively lengthy journey (Toombs, 1995, p.13). Hence the temporal scale of her narrative underwent a significant change. Journeys which had hitherto taken little time, now took up a great deal of time.

Suppose this example of the change in Toombs' narrative is factored in to her life as a whole, i.e. not simply in terms of the journey from her office to her classroom. For example, consider the changes in the time it takes, say, to get out of bed in the morning, to get changed, to shower, prepare breakfast, to do some shopping, to visit friends. Toombs indicates how the development of MS had ramifications for the timescale needed to engage in these typical, everyday tasks.

So, given that time is plausibly construed as a structuring concept in the narratives of persons, and given that temporal relations are radically affected by certain types of disabilities (especially, but not solely, motor disabilities), and given the distinction between objective and subjective time, it is plausible to claim that disablement results in a change in the nature of the narrative of a person, a change which it is reasonable to describe as metaphysically deep, indeed, as identity-constituting. It is a change which will figure in an answer to the question 'who?' when this is posed of Toombs.

With regard to embodiment, as seen, Toombs observes that one's body now seems to be an obstacle to the projects of the self, inhibiting the pursuit of those projects. At one level, the sense in which the body is an obstacle is revealed in the performance of actions which, hitherto, one performed without thinking. Actions such as reaching for a cup or stirring sugar into a hot drink become problematic, in that one now has to concentrate upon these in a way which one needn't do prior to the development of the disease.

At another level, actions such as going swimming, jogging or cycling become impossible. And acts such as visiting a café or a relative are also made problematic (e.g. due to need for ramps etc.).

With regard to one's self-conception, the view one has of the kind of person one aspires to be, Toombs describes how this too can be jeopardised by MS. Obviously, aspirations to be an athlete or any physically demanding roles are at best seriously jeopardised. And, again as with MS, aspirations which involve long periods of concentrated study are also jeopardised.

It should be noted that this account of identity dovetails rather neatly with the theory of disablement endorsed in Part One. In that, recall, the question of whether or not a person is disabled hinges upon the pursuance of their vital goals. If, having developed MS,

Toombs judges that her ability to pursue her vital goals has been compromised, she may well judge that she has a disability. So a revision in her self-conception occurs (indicated in the fact that she opted to become a part-time as opposed to a full-time lecturer). So a key moment in her narrative is this revision of self-conception, and the explanation for the revision is her development of MS, a condition she regards as disabling.

Relatedly, since one's self-conception will be called into question by conditions such as MS, or by the kind of accident which beset Morris, so too will one's self-project. (Murphy refers to his acquisition of an 'embattled identity' (Murphy, 1987, p.89).) The mini-projects one has which are oriented towards fulfilment of one's self-conception may be jeopardised by chronic illness or disability. In her own case, Toombs describes how her goals changed as a direct consequence of her condition. She considered full-time lecturing to present too many challenges to her, given her MS. So she opted for a part-time lecturing position.

Toombs' analysis illustrates the very significant changes in the life of the person that follow from the development of a chronic illness. These are changes in the way the world is experienced, and in the significance or purpose of one's life (i.e. in the way one's life is lived and the meaning of it for one). In the same vein, Murphy writes (1987, p.77) 'Disability is not simply a physical affair; it is our ontology, a condition of our being in the world'. Also, 'I had changed in my own mind, in my self-image, and in the basic condition of my existence' (Murphy, 1987, p.73).

So far in our discussion of the concepts which are claimed here to 'structure' narratives, no mention has yet been made of other persons; *their* bodies, *their* self-conceptions, *their* values. Yet it is plain that these will also be crucial. At an obvious level, family members, loved ones, those for whom one has great respect (one's teachers, great artists, sports persons and so on) are all plausible candidates for inclusion in the fleshing out of a narrative.

But at a deeper level, other persons bear upon the structuring concepts identified above. As we heard in our discussion of the work of Taylor, our thoughts recruit concepts from our linguistic communities, and our patterns of interactions with others are shaped in part by value-laden and culturally variable notions such as embarrassment, shame, or pride. So at this deeper level, the narratives of persons are constrained and constituted by relations with other persons. This is most evident in the categories of self-conception and self-project.

This value-component to the narratives of persons has particular relevance to the area of disablement. For, as argued above, it is plausible to claim that people with disabilities are accorded a moral status which is less than that accorded to those considered 'able' (what we described earlier as the 'low moral status' claim). This view can be articulated within Taylor's conception of 'moral space' (Taylor, 1989, Chapter 2). Roughly, his claim is that judgements concerning what is good or bad, in moral terms, occur within a general framework and represent certain patterns of evaluations. For example, from within a religious moral framework, an action may be considered good if it is in concordance with what is deemed good according to that religion (e.g. being merciful, or charitable). A grip can be got upon the spatial metaphor by thinking of, say, the notions of good and what is morally worthy as being at one 'region' of moral space, and what is considered bad, undesirable or unworthy at a different region of moral space. If the low moral status claim is accepted, it can be argued that the region of moral space within which disablement is typically conceived of, is a region in which those things which are not valued, and which may even be disvalued, are (metaphorically) 'located'. In fact, this 'disvaluing' is well-documented (*see* especially Morris, 1991, pp.39–63 (e.g. p.43); Alderson, 2001). All the considerations recruited in support of the low moral status claim bear this out.

If this proposal is accepted, at least two points seem to follow. The first is that interactions between people with (especially visible) disabilities and those who are non-disabled are likely to be affected by the conception of disability prevalent in a particular culture (again, *see* previous references). So the character of such interactions is affected by the fact that one of the participants has a disability. This is borne out by at least some empirical evidence. For example, one reason offered for performing cosmetic surgery on people with Down's syndrome is that it helps to pre-empt initial, typically negative, responses from potential employers (*see* Edwards, 1996). Also, a disabled person interviewed by Morris described how she responded to people who stared at her, she would shout at them 'What are you staring at?' (Morris, 1991, p.26). And other disabled people interviewed by Morris report that their interactions with others and their self-conceptions are partly determined by the fact of their disablement (*see also* Murphy, 1987, pp.74–5; Toombs, 1995, p.16).

Second, if the negative evaluation of disablement is accepted (i.e. if it is accepted that such negative evaluations are widespread), then it seems likely that the self-conception of people will similarly be affected by this. Hence the evaluative component present in all narratives is likely to be reflected in the narratives of people with disabilities, as this is constructed from the first-person perspective. Moreover, given acceptance of the claim that narratives are constructed from both third- and first-person perspectives, it follows that the moral status accorded to people with disabilities will again be reflected in the narratives of disabled people (again, *see* Alderson, 2001).

Finally, on this general topic, it is worth describing a further point made by Toombs (also, Jonas 1974). She argues that the very fact of using a wheelchair for mobility has a deep effect upon both her self-conception and the conceptions of her held by others. The reason she puts forward is that 'upright posture is directly related to autonomy' (Toombs, 1995, p.16). In a similar vein, Sacks writes: 'erectness [in posture] is moral, existential, no less than physical' (Sacks, 1984, p.98). And Murphy writes of his sense of lowered self-worth (1987) which he attributed to his use of a wheelchair.

Toombs points out that when infants learn to walk and to stand this is considered a key moment in their development. It heralds the transition to an autonomous, independent agent. So there is a clear value-element to posture, and, at least according to Toombs (and others), people who are not able to walk independently are considered not to be fully autonomous. In support of this she goes on to describe how, if she is in her wheelchair she is not addressed directly but 'through' her husband, and gives numerous examples of related types of interactions in which it seems plain that she is not regarded as a full moral agent (*see also* Murphy, 1987, p.102, and the BBC Radio programme ironically titled *Does he take sugar?*, www.bbc.co.uk/ouch).

So far, then, we have identified certain concepts claimed here to structure the narratives of persons (those of time, space, embodiment, self-conception, self-project). And a case has been made to indicate how disablement may be viewed through each of these structuring concepts.

We have seen how from the perspective of the person concerned, the experience of disablement is manifested in significant impacts upon the nature of the narratives of selves with disabilities, when this is considered from the first-person perspective and in terms of the concepts identified here as structuring concepts.

So, in the specific case of a person such as Toombs or Jenny Morris (or RF Murphy etc. etc.) their identity will be given by a narrative, one which answers the question 'who?'. As described above, disablement is very likely to feature in their respective narratives. This is due to its impact upon space as lived, time as lived, embodiment, self-conception and self-project. Their respective bodies will provide a 'site of narration' (to use Kerby's expression (1991, p.4)). Their narratives will be dependent upon their social context, the language available within it, and its value-orientation. Hence their identities, as with the identities of all humans, will be infused with characteristics external to them (e.g. the types of phenomena just given). So, contrary to ontological individualism, their identities will exhibit ontological anti-individualism in the sense that their identities presuppose and require the specification of phenomena beyond their bodies.

If the above account of identity is accepted, it can be seen how disablement is an 'identity-constituting' feature for those people who acquire disabilities during their lifetime. The completion of the five structuring concepts of a narrative will probably include reference to disablement. This is due to the impact of disablement on the five aspects of personal existence.

Nothing has been said so far about people who are born with disabling conditions – with congenital disabilities such as cystic fibrosis, spina bifida and Down's syndrome. How can the approach to questions of identity just sketched cope with these?

Consider Down's syndrome first. It was observed above that we are not the authors of our own narratives; such narratives are constrained by third-person considerations. In the case of Down's syndrome these include the place in moral space accorded to intellectually disabled people; this was evidenced in the existence and expansion of prenatal screening programmes and the contemplation of plastic surgery for people with Down's syndrome. With cystic fibrosis, again it seems reasonable to claim this will figure in the narrative of the person concerned. The effects upon lifestyle, due to respiratory problems associated with the condition, seem likely to impact upon the self-conception of the person, to have a limiting effect upon this. And lastly with regard to spina bifida, the approach described here could not determine in advance of the person's life whether or not this would feature in the person's narrative. It would depend upon the severity of the condition for the person concerned. If there is an impact in any of the five aspects, then it will feature in the narrative of the person. It should be remembered that, in situations where the person is capable of expressing a view, strictly speaking, the question of that person's disablement is not independent of their opinion. This holds true for both 'acquired' and genetically based impairments.

Summary

The theory of personal identity just sketched allows that contingent properties can figure in the identity conditions of persons. As noted, it is a position partly inspired by some work of Ricoeur. Thus in relation to, say Jenny Morris or SK Toombs, one gives their identity by answering this question (i.e. the question 'who?'). The proposal advanced here is that an answer to the question 'who?' would require the giving of a life story, or an extract of a life story: of a narrative which describes a life. Answering the question 'who?' demands the provision of an extract from a narrative, since the mere giving of a proper name does not sufficiently answer the question.

So this position allows that, due to the extent of the changes in the lives of Toombs and Morris brought about by disability, a change in the nature of the person occurs. Disablement can be counted among the causes of that change, bearing in mind that any such claim is constrained by the opinion of the person whose narrative is under discussion. But there is no change in subject, no change in numerical identity; further identifying features are added to the narrative.

The narrative of the person includes descriptions of the person's pursuance of a self-project. Hence Toombs' narrative will be likely to include her philosophical aspirations and achievements, plus the story of her MS. (This latter will be 'emplotted' (Ricoeur, 1992, p.147), i.e. woven into her narrative.)

As stated, the account of identity being outlined here is that of narrative identity. In this, one's pursuance of a self-project is described in a narrative. In answering the question 'who?' one relates what has happened to a person and what a person does. Of course this can be done by the person concerned or by an observer. A narrative will comprise elements from both first- and third-person perspectives. And, of course, such descriptions (of what has happened to x and of what x has done) will themselves be in narrative form. They'll be events or sequences of events given in narrative form, with beginnings, middles and ends. In fact the very development of disability or chronic illness will probably be understood in narrative terms, e.g. as bad luck or as punishment from God.

Morris' disability and Toombs' MS seem plausible candidates for inclusion in their respective narratives, since these events have such a far-reaching impact upon the five aspects of human existence mentioned earlier. (As we saw, Morris says she has acquired an identity as a disabled woman.) Hence in this sense one is doing justice to the idea that a radical change in the person has occurred: e.g. in relation to the changes in the five dimensions listed above, while at the same time recognising that contingent features of a person can figure in their identity conditions. These (identity conditions) are specified in the person's narrative.

So the identity of Toombs and Morris is described by a narrative. The content of the narrative will be contingent, but certain structures will not be, specifically those relating to the five structuring concepts of personal existence.

The expressivist objection

The work just done on the identity claim paves the way for a brief assessment of the objection to the practice of PGD outlined at the start of this part of the book. The view that the practice of PGD and termination sends a negative message to disabled people is, apparently, commonly held (*see* Parens and Asch, 2000, and the Disabled Peoples' International (DPI) statement overleaf). And it is sometimes termed 'the expressivist argument': the argument that PGD (with consequent termination of pregnancy on grounds of disability) sends a negative message to currently living disabled people (Buchanan, 1996).

It seems to me that the basis of the argument stems from a view of the relationship between disablement and identity, such that the latter can be identity-constituting. This possibility is rarely taken seriously by critics of proponents of the expressivist objection. But in our discussion we have shown how disablement can be identity-constituting. So what implications will this have for the force of the expressivist argument?

In his arguments in support of prenatal screening for genetic anomalies associated with disabilities, John Harris offers the following observation. He writes:

> I just do not believe that attempts to remove or pre-empt dysfunction or disability constitute discrimination against the disabled as a group, anymore than medical treatment of disease discriminates against the sick as a group (Harris, 2000, p.96).[1]

However, as noted many people with disabilities hold the view that selective abortion on grounds of disability does convey a message, or otherwise imply, that it would have been better had they not been born. For example, the Disabled Peoples' International (DPI) statement on 'the new genetics' claims that:

> The underlying reason for pre-natal screening and testing is the elimination of the impaired foetus. This sends a discriminatory message to say that disabled people's lives are not worth living or worthy of support (DPI, 2000, p.7).

The claim that prenatal screening 'sends' such a message has become known as the 'expressivist argument', a term coined by Buchanan (1996). The position espoused by the DPI displays commitment to the expressivist argument.

Against the expressivist argument a view exactly like that put forward by Harris is typically advanced. As we heard, this is that reducing the incidence of disabling traits no more sends a negative message to disabled people than reducing the incidence of flu sends a negative message to flu sufferers.

One commentator Baily, a woman who underwent amniocentesis, says of the expressivist argument that it 'only makes sense if people with disabilities are their disabilities' (in Parens and Asch, 2000, p.68). And it is this observation which goes to the heart of the matter in my view.

Commentators who cannot see the force of the expressivist objec-

---

[1]It is interesting to juxtapose this claim with the earlier claim, quoted above and repeated here from Harris: '...anyone who thinks that the detection of handicap in the foetus is a good reason for abortion, must accept that such an individual is, or will become, less valuable than one without such a handicap, less valuable because less worth saving or less entitled to life' (Harris, 1985, p.7).

tion see no relevant difference between reduction of the incidence of disability and reduction of the incidence of any disease. Thus just as reducing the incidence of flu can only be a desirable end, so too must reducing the incidence of a condition such as Down's syndrome or cystic fibrosis. For, in the eyes of such commentators (not implausibly) just as there is no question of a person being defined as a 'flu sufferer', there is no question of a person being defined in terms of their disability (*see* e.g. Buchanan, 1996, p.32). Such commentators take illnesses such as flu to be contingent to a person's identity and they extend this 'contingency' view to disabilities.

But as we have seen, many reject such a 'contingency' view of disabilities. And we have shown how disabling traits may, in fact, be at least partly identity-constituting: hence, a description of the identity conditions of at least some groups of disabled people would include reference to their disabilities.

However, the wrongness of termination of pregnancy following diagnosis of disabling traits in the foetus still does not follow. To see this, recall that the main objection to the practice of prenatal screening from the perspective of the DPI is the discriminatory message such a practice conveys to the effect that 'disabled people's lives are not worth living or worthy of support'. In other words, the moral wrongness of the practice stems from the harmful effects it has. These harmful effects include, most saliently, the offence and hurt felt by people currently living with the kinds of disabling traits screened for in the practice of prenatal screening.

But there are three grounds for resisting the expressivist objection, even if one allows that disabling traits can be identity-constituting.

First, the wrong done by prenatal screening is that of the hurt or offence that practice conveys to existing disabled people. (Since abortion is not objectionable *per se* to members of the DPI.) But of course it does not follow from this that it is right to place the obligation not to harm others above the right to have one's own reproductive autonomy respected. One is obliged to take into account consequences of one's actions which might harm others, but it does not follow that those harms count for more than the suppression of one's free choice. One might choose to be a meat eater knowing this will offend vegetarians and lead to some harm to animals. But it does not follow that the harms to these other parties should 'trump' one's own autonomous choices. Or one may choose to have an abortion in the knowledge that this will offend pro-life groups, but it does not follow that the offence caused to these groups outweighs one's right to make such a choice. Exactly the same response can be made against the expressivist objection.

So, from the moral perspective, accepting the identity claim, the expressivist objection to prenatal screening is vulnerable to objection. It appears to require moral agents to place the obligations not to harm others above their wishes to enact their autonomous choices, and their choices to avoid avoidable harms. But in this case there is no reason why they should so place the interests of others above their own interests in having their reproductive autonomy respected.

Second, one can consistently hold two views: (a) prenatal screening is justified; and (b) disabled people should be supported, and certainly should not be abandoned on grounds of disability. Thus, the 'loss of support' need not follow from the continued practice of prenatal screening.

Third, acceptance of the expressivist objection seems to lead to a *reductio ad absurdum* to be described now. On the face of it, it looks as though the objection implies that any means of reducing the incidence of disablement is objectionable. For of course any such reduction brings with it a reduction in the numbers of disabled people.

This objection will apply in the case of disabilities which have a genetic origin (Down's syndrome, cystic fibrosis etc). But also, perhaps counter-intuitively, it will apply in cases where disability is caused in some other way, e.g. by illness or physical trauma (as in the case of Christopher Reeve for example).

In either of these types of cases in removing the disability one thereby reduces the numbers of disabled persons, and 'sends a message' to people who have the relevant disabling condition. This is so even if the person themself decides to have their disability removed, e.g. by surgical intervention to remove deafness or blindness or paraplegia and so on.

So the expressivist objection seems to have the implication that it is wrong both first, to seek to prevent any form of disability, and second, to cure or 'put right' any existing disability.

If it is true that the objection has these implications, then some might justifiably regard the expressivist objection as vulnerable to criticism on the grounds that its acceptance leads to absurd consequences, specifically, the consequence that it is wrong to rectify or even to seek to prevent the incidence of disabling conditions. Thus, even if an 'identity claim' is accepted to the effect that disabling traits can be identity-constituting, and thus are not analogous to flu and other illnesses, the wrongness of prenatal genetic diagnosis need not follow.

Conclusion

In this part of our discussion we began by looking at the point of examining the relationship between disablement and the person. As shown, differing philosophical accounts imply differing views of disablement. An emergentist theory of the person was supported. After a brief discussion of the person/human being distinction, the question of the relationship between disablement and identity was discussed. A theory of personal identity was developed, according to which disablement can be identity-constituting. The discussion closed with a brief assessment of the implications of this for the expressivist argument. It was seen that even if disablement is identity-constituting, the expressivist argument is not a compelling one.

Conclusion

As mentioned in the introduction, the topics discussed in the three parts of this book may appear unrelated, or related only tenuously. But this is not so. The concept of narrative provides a unifying theme which can fruitfully be brought to bear on the three parts of our discussion. To see this, recall that in Part One we offered general support for the account of disablement provided by Lennart Nordenfelt. In this, as we saw, the question of whether a person has an impairment can, in principle, be answered without any reference to the view of the person concerned. But this is not so in relation to the question of whether or not the person is disabled. If the person is capable of expressing a view, then the answer to the question must pay close attention to, and give great weight to, the view of the person concerned. If they say they can attain their vital goals, and if they can indeed attain them, and their necessary conditions, they are not disabled according to Nordenfelt's theory. The vital goals of a person will be goals which provide an overriding purpose for a person. They are aims which, in that person's eyes, are central components of their life. Put in narrative terms, they are key components of the person's self-conception. If the presence of impairment, in concert with external factors such as absence of social support or wheelchair-inaccessible public transport systems, obstructs a person's pursuance of their self-conception, they are plausibly regarded as disabled. Determination of whether they actually are disabled, as we saw, must pay great weight to the view of the person concerned, the person whose disability is in question. So it can be seen that the idea of a vital goal dovetails with the idea of a self-conception. A goal is 'vital' to a person since it connects up with their view of the kind of person they aspire to be, of the kind of life they wish to lead, of the kind of narrative they want to exemplify. It is evident, then, that the theory of disablement championed in Part One is itself parasitic upon the notion of a narrative. For the question of whether or not a person is disabled is inseparable from the question of whether that person can lead the kind of life they wish to lead.

So much, then, for the way in which the concerns of Part One connect up with the idea of a narrative. What of the concerns of Part Two, regarding the grounds for terminations of pregnancy when allegedly disabling genetic traits (impairments) are diagnosed in the foetus. The way this can be explained in narrative terms is as follows. When considering a termination, the woman inevitably considers the effects of either terminating the pregnancy or continuing with it, in terms of its effects upon her capacity to pursue her self-conception. If she envisages that the birth of a disabled child will severely jeopardise that pursuit then, plainly, she is more likely to opt for termination. This was evident in the actual case we analysed in Part Two, that of Emma Loach and her family. Emma considers the effects of having a child with Down's syndrome upon her capacity to pursue her own self-conception. She also considers the effects on the lives of her partner Elliot and son Samuel. In each case she is thinking of the ways in which having a child with Down's syndrome will affect the narratives of the people closest to her. As we saw, her judgement is that their self-projects will be severely jeopardised if she proceeds with the pregnancy. And also, of course, she considers the likely narrative of the future child. Based upon the information she was provided with, she concludes that the narrative which the future child will exemplify will be a severely impoverished one, filled with suffering and disvalued characteristics such as excessive dependence upon others. Hence, here again we can see the concept of a narrative as unifying both the themes within Part Two, and those of Part One in which, as shown, the idea of disability is intimately linked to that of narrative, as though the narrative of a disabled person is somehow inevitably a 'damaged' narrative in the sense that disability or impairment will inevitably pollute a person's capacity to lead a good life. It was argued in Part Two that such views are almost certainly false.

It is in Part Three where the most explicit use of narrative is made. Here an attempt is made to develop a theory of narrative identity. It adopts a novel strategy in trying to do this, appealing to the five structuring concepts of personal existence. It was explained in Part Three how acquired disability could not credibly be 'identity constituting' in traditional approaches to the problem of personal identity. But the narrative approach allows room for acquired disabilities insofar as any changes to the body which have deep ramifications for the person's narrative, specifically their self-conception and self-project, are credibly regarded as identity constituting. Thus, it is plain that the concept of narrative can be put to good use in this context too.

So that, in crude outline, is how the three parts of the discussion can be unified by exploitation of the idea of narrative. The use of it in Part Three is probably the most ambitious since that attempts to develop a novel account of personal identity. But if asked to highlight one particular component of the book as being of especial importance I would suggest it is the discussion of disability and the good life. This shows, to my mind, that disability is not incompatible with leading a good human life, and, especially given external support, need not impugn a person's capacity to lead a maximally good life.

References

Alderson P (2001) Down's syndrome: cost, quality and value of life. *Social Science and Medicine.* **53**: 627–38.

Americans with Disabilities Act (1990) Pub. L No. 101–336, 42 USC 12101 *et seq.*

Aristotle (translated by JAK Thomson, 1953) *Nichomachean Ethics.* Penguin, Harmondsworth.

Baily MA (2000) Why I had amniocentesis. In: E Parens and A Asch (eds) *Prenatal Testing and Disability Rights.* Georgetown University Press, Georgetown, pp. 64–71.

Baker LR (2000) *Persons and Bodies, a Constitution View.* Cambridge University Press, Cambridge.

Bauby J-D (1997) *The Diving Bell and the Butterfly.* Fourth Estate, London.

Beauchamp TL and Childress JF (2001) *Principles of Biomedical Ethics* (5e). Oxford University Press, Oxford.

Belshaw C (2000) Identity and disability. *Journal of Applied Philosophy.* **17**: 263–76.

Benner P (2000) The role of embodiment, emotion and lifeworld for rationality and agency in nursing practice. *Nursing Philosophy.* **1**: 5–19.

Bickenbach JE, Chatterji S, Badley EM and Ustun TB (1999) Models of disablement, universalism and the ICIDH. *Social Science and Medicine.* **48**: 1173–87.

Boorse C (1975) On the distinction between disease and illness. *Philosophy and Public Affairs.* **5**: 49–68.

Broad CD (1929) *Mind and its Place in Nature.* Routledge and Kegan Paul, London.

Brock D (1993) Quality of life measures in health care and medical ethics. In: M Nussbaum and A Sen (eds) *The Quality of Life.* Clarendon Press, Oxford, pp. 95–132.

Buchanan A (1996) Genetic manipulation and the morality of inclusion. *Social Philosophy and Policy.* **13**: 18–46.

Burt C (1937) *The Subnormal Mind* (2e). Oxford University Press, London.

Campbell J (2003) Choose life. *The Guardian.* 26 August.

Churchland P (1979) *Scientific Realism and the Plasticity of Mind.* Cambridge University Press, Cambridge.

Dennett D (1981) *Brainstorms.* Harvester Press, Brighton.

Department of Health (2003) *Our Inheritance, Our Future. Realising the potential of genetics in the NHS.* The Stationery Office, London.

Descartes R (1637/1954) Discourse on method. In: PT Geach and EA Anscombe (edited and translated) *Philosophical Writings.* Nelson and Sons, London, pp. 5–57.

Descartes R (1641/1954) Meditations on first philosophy. In: PT Geach and E Anscombe (edited and translated) *Philosophical Writings.* Nelson and Sons, London, pp. 59–124.

Descartes R (1649/1969) The passions of the soul part 1. In: MD Wilson (ed.) *The Essential Descartes.* Mentor Books, London, pp. 353–68.

Disability Discrimination Act (1995) The Stationery Office, London.

Disabled Peoples' International (DPI) (2000) *Disabled People Speak on the New Genetics*. Disabled Peoples International Europe, London.

Edwards SD (1996) Plastic surgery and individuals with Down's syndrome. In: I de Beaufort, M Hilhorst and S Holm (eds) *The Eye of the Beholder, Ethics and Medical Change of Appearance*. Scandinavian University Press, Oslo, pp. 26–33.

Edwards SD (1997a) The moral status of intellectually disabled individuals. *Journal of Medicine and Philosophy*. **22**: 29–42.

Edwards SD (1997b) Dismantling the disability/handicap distinction. *Journal of Medicine and Philosophy*. **22**: 589–606.

Edwards SD (1998) The body as object versus the body as subject: the case of disability. *Medicine, Health Care and Philosophy*. **1**: 47–56.

Elster J and Hylland A (eds) (1986) *Foundations of Social Choice Theory*. Cambridge University Press, Cambridge.

Elster J and Roemer JE (eds) (1991) *Interpersonal Comparisons of Well-being*. Cambridge University Press, Cambridge.

Ferguson PM, Gartner A, Lipsky DK *et al.* (2000) The experience of disability in families: a synthesis of research and parent narratives. In: E Parens and A Asch (eds) *Prenatal Testing and Disability Rights*. Georgetown University Press, Georgetown, pp. 72–94.

Finkelstein V (1993) The commonality of disability. In: J Swain, V Finkelstein, S French and M Oliver (eds) *Disabling Barriers, Enabling Environments*. Sage, London, pp. 9–16.

Gadow S (1982) Body and self. In: V Kestenbaum (ed.) *The Humanity of the Ill, Phenomenological Perspectives*. University of Tennessee Press, Knoxville, pp. 86–100.

Gauthier D (1986) The liberal individual. In: S Avineri and A de-Shalit (eds) *Communitarianism and Individualism*. Oxford University Press, Oxford, pp. 151–64.

Goodin RE (1986) Laundering preferences. In: J Elster and A Hylland (eds) *Foundations of Social Choice Theory*. Cambridge University Press, Cambridge, pp. 75–101.

Greaves D (1996) *Mystery in Western Medicine*. Ashgate, Aldershot.

Greenhalgh T and Hurwitz B (1998) *Narrative-based Medicine*. BMJ Publishing, London.

Griffin J (1986) *Well-being, Its Meaning, Measurement and Moral Importance*. Clarendon Press, Oxford.

Hare RM (1974) The abnormal child: moral dilemmas of doctors and parents. In: H Kuhse and P Singer (eds) *Bioethics, an anthology*. Blackwell, Oxford, pp. 269–72.

Harris J (1985) *The Value of Life*. Routledge, London.

Harris J (1998) *Clones, Genes and Immortality*. Oxford University Press, Oxford.

Harris J (2000) Is there a coherent social conception of disability? *Journal of Medical Ethics*. **26**: 95–100.

Heaton-Ward WA and Wiley Y (1984) *Mental Handicap* (5e). Wright, Bristol.

Human Fertilisation and Embryology Act (1990) The Stationery Office, London.

Human Genetics Commission (2004) *Choosing the Future: genetics and reproductive decision making*. Department of Health, London.

Husserl E (1913/1962) *Ideas*. Collier Books, New York.

Johnson HB (2003) Unspeakable conversations. *New York Times*. 16 February.

Jonas H (1974) *Philosophical Essays, from Ancient Creed to Technological Man*. University of Chicago Press, Chicago.

Kant I (1781/1929) *Critique of Pure Reason*. Macmillan, London.

Kerby AP (1991) *Narrative and the Self*. Indiana University Press, Bloomington.

Kim J (1995) Physicalism in the philosophy of mind. In: T Honderich (ed.) *A Companion to Philosophy*. Oxford University Press, Oxford, pp. 679–80.

Kleinman A (1988) *Illness Narratives, Suffering, Healing and the Human Condition*. Basic Books, New York.

Kripke S (1981) *Naming and Necessity*. Blackwell, Oxford.

Kuhse H and Singer P (1985) *Should the Baby Live?* Oxford University Press, Oxford.

Loach E (2003) The hardest thing I have ever done. *The Guardian*. 31 May.

Lonsdale S (1990) *Women and Disability*. Macmillan, London.

Lukes S (1973) *Individualism*. Blackwell, Oxford.

Macdonald C (1989) *Mind–Brain Identity Theories*. Routledge, London.

MacIntyre A (1981) *After Virtue, a Study in Moral Theory*. Duckworth, London.

MacIntyre A (1999) *Dependent Rational Animals*. Duckworth, London.

Mason JK and McCall Smith RA (1994) *Law and Medical Ethics*. Butterworths, London.

McGinn C (1982) *The Character of Mind*. Oxford University Press, Oxford.

Merleau-Ponty M (translated by C Smith) (1945/1962) *The Phenomenology of Perception*. Routledge, London.

Mill JS (1859/1962) *On Liberty*. In: M Warnock (ed.) *Utilitarianism*. Fontana Press, London, pp. 126–250.

Mill JS (1861/1962) *Utilitarianism*. In: M Warnock (ed.) *Utilitarianism*. Fontana Press, London, pp. 251–321.

Morris J (1991) *Pride Against Prejudice*. Women's Press, London.

Mundy I (2002) A world of their own. *Washington Post*. 27 March.

Munhall S and Swift A (1992) *Liberals and Communitarians*. Blackwell, Oxford.

Murphy RF (1987) *The Body Silent*. Phoenix House, London.

Nordenfelt L (1983/1997) *On Disabilities and Their Classification*. University of Linkopping, Linkopping.

Nordenfelt L (1993a) On the notions of disability and handicap. *Social Welfare*. **2**: 17–24.

Nordenfelt L (1993b) *Quality of Life, Health and Happiness*. Avebury, Aldershot.

Nordenfelt L (1995) *On the Nature of Health*. Kluwer, Dordrecht.

Nordenfelt L (1997) The importance of a disability/handicap distinction. *Journal of Medicine and Philosophy*. **22**: 607–22.

Nordenfelt L (1999) On disability and illness, a reply to Edwards. *Theoretical Medicine*. **20**: 181–9.

Nordenfelt L (2000) *Action, Ability and Health*. Kluwer, Dordrecht.

Nordenfelt L (2001) *Health, Science and Ordinary Language*. Rodopi, Amsterdam.

Nozick R (1974) *Anarchy, State and Utopia*. Basic Books, New York.

Nozick R (1981) *Philosophical Explanations*. Oxford University Press, Oxford.

Nussbaum M (1988) Nature, function, and capability: Aristotle on political distribution. In: J Annas (ed.) *Oxford Studies in Ancient Philosophy*. Clarendon, Oxford, pp. 145–84.

Nussbaum M and Sen A (eds) (1993) *The Quality of Life*. Clarendon Press, Oxford.

Oliver M (1990) *The Politics of Disablement*. Macmillan, London.

Parens E and Asch A (eds) (2000) *Prenatal Testing and Disability Rights*. Georgetown University Press, Georgetown.

Parfit R (1984) *Reasons and Persons*. Oxford University Press, Oxford.

Persson I (1995) Genetic therapy, identity and person-regarding reasons. *Bioethics*. 9: 16–31.

Plato (translated by D Lee, 1974) *The Republic*. Penguin, London.

Rawls J (1970) *A Theory of Justice*. Oxford University Press, Oxford.

Rée J (1999) *I See a Voice*. Flamingo, London.

Reinders H (2000) *The Future of the Disabled in Liberal Society: an ethical analysis*. University of Notre Dame Press, Notre Dame.

Ricoeur P (1991) Narrative identity. *Philosophy Today*. **Spring:** 73–81.

Ricoeur P (1992) *Oneself as Another*. University of Chicago Press, Chicago.

Sacks O (1984) *A Leg to Stand On*. Picador, London.

Sacks O (1989) *Seeing Voices*. Picador, London.

Sacks O (1995) *An Anthropologist on Mars*. Picador, London.

Schectman H (1996) *The Constitution of Selves*. Cornell University Press, Ithaca.

Sedgwick P (1982) *Psychopolitics*. Pluto Press, London.

Sen A (1993) Capability and well-being. In: M Nussbaum and A Sen (eds) *The Quality of Life*. Clarendon Press, Oxford, pp. 30–53.

Shoemaker S and Swinburne R (1984) *Personal Identity*. Blackwell, Oxford.

Singer P (1993) *Practical Ethics* (2e). Cambridge University Press, Cambridge.

Smart JJC (1959) Sensations and brain processes. In: C Borst (ed.) (1970) *Mind/Brain Identity Theory*. Macmillan, London, pp. 52–66.

Swain J, Finkelstein V, French S and Oliver M (eds) (1993) *Disabling Barriers, Enabling Environments*. Sage, London.

Taylor C (1989) *Sources of the Self*. Cambridge University Press, Cambridge.

Tooley M (1972) Abortion and infanticide. *Philosophy and Public Affairs*. **2:** 37–65.

Toombs SK (1993) *The Meaning of Illness, a Phenomenological Account of the Different Perspectives of the Physician and Patient*. Kluwer, Dordrecht.

Toombs SK (1995) Sufficient unto the day: a life with multiple sclerosis. In: SK Toombs, D Barnard and RA Carson (eds) *Chronic Illness, from Experience to Policy*. Indiana University Press, Indianapolis, pp. 3–22.

Union of the Physically Impaired Against Segregation (UPIAS) (1975) *Fundamental Principles of Disability*. UPIAS, London.

van Hooft S (1995) *Caring, an Essay in the Philosophy of Ethics*. Colorado University Press, Boulder.

Veatch RM (1986) *The Foundations of Justice*. Oxford University Press, Oxford.

Wendell S (1996) *The Rejected Body, Feminist Philosophical Reflections on Disability*. Routledge, London.

Wilkes KV (1993) *Personal Identity Without Thought Experiments*. Clarendon Press, Oxford.

Williams B (1973) *Problems of the Self*. Cambridge University Press, Cambridge.

Williams B (1978) *Descartes: the project of pure enquiry.* Pelican, Harmondsworth.

Wilson E (1979) *The Mental as Physical.* Routledge, London.

World Health Organization (WHO) (1946) *Constitution.* WHO, Geneva.

World Health Organization (WHO) (1980/1993) *International Classification of Impairments, Disabilities and Handicaps.* WHO, Geneva.

World Health Organization (WHO) (2001) *The International Classification of Functioning, Disability and Health.* WHO, Geneva.

Index

abilities
  cf. capacities 13
  defining disablement 6
ableism 38–40
abortion 8, 9, 53–9, 111–12
Aristotelean *good human life* concept
  77–81

benefits, social 8
biomedical model of disease 17
Blunkett, David 45

Campbell, Jane 84–5
capacities, cf. abilities 13
Cartesian dualism 99–104
causes
  disability 16
  handicap 16
Churchland, Paul 92
classificatory systems
  ICF 32–40
  ICIDH 9–19
Conservative party 'core beliefs' 86
contingency 49
criticisms
  ICIDH 13–19
  responses to 44–8

deafness, preference satisfaction theory
  70
defining
  disability 11, 19–24, 30–4
  handicap 11–12, 23
  impairment 10–11, 13, 19–22, 32–3
  participation restriction 34
dependence 55–6
disability
  causes 16
  defining 11, 19–24, 30–4

  vs. handicap 16–18
Disabled Peoples' International (DPI)
  140
disablement
  emergentism 106–10
  identity and 97–110, 113–19,
    119–23
  identity-constituting feature 137
  narrative identity 119–23, 137
  personal identity 97–110, 113–19
  structuring concepts 130–8
discrimination 38–40
  justice principle 38–40
disease, cf. illness 47–8
disvalued states 44–7
domestic/public spheres, *good human life*
  concept 65–6
Down's syndrome 11, 51–2, 54–9
  hedonistic theory 60–4
  maximising approach 67–8, 89
  narrative identity 137
  objective goods theory 81–4, 90–1
  preference satisfaction theory 69,
    72–7
DPI (Disabled Peoples' International) 140
dualism
  Cartesian 99–104
  individualism 100–4
  philosophical theory 98–104

embodiment, personal existence 126–8
emergentism
  disablement 106–10
  MS 108–9
  philosophical theory 98, 106–10
  sensory disabilities 107–8
  syndrome Z 107
Emma Loach 54–9, 63–4, 72–7, 81–4,
  93–4

EPC (essential properties constraint) 118–20
epidemiological perspective 18
essential properties constraint (EPC) 118–20
ethical individualism 100–4
expressivist objection 139–43

fair societies 85–6
features, disablement 5–7
foetuses *see* pregnancy

good human life concept 53–95
    hedonistic theory 59–68
    length of life 60–2
    maximising approach 66–8, 87–94
    objective goods theory 77–94
    preference satisfaction theory 68–77
    public/domestic spheres 65–6
    threshold approach 87–8

handicap
    causes 16
    defining 11–12, 23
    vs. disability 16–18
Harris, Prof. John 140
    defining disability 30–2
    pregnancy termination 111–12
hearing-related preferences, preference satisfaction theory 70
hedonistic theory, *good human life* concept 59–68
human beings, and persons 109
Human Fertilisation and Embryology Act (1990) 111
hypothetical syndrome Z 53–9, 60

ICF *see* International Classification of Functioning, Disability and Health
ICIDH *see* International Classification of Impairments, Disabilities and Handicaps
identity
    disablement and 97–110, 113–19
    narrative identity 119–23, 137
    structuring concepts 123–30

identity-constituting feature, disablement 137
illness, cf. disease 47–8
impairment, defining 10–11, 13, 19–22, 32–3
independence 55–6
individualism
    dualism 100–4
    ethical 100–4
    ontological 100–4
intellectual disabilities, preference satisfaction theory 71–2, 90
interdependence 55–6
International Classification of Functioning, Disability and Health (ICF) 32–40
    cf. ICIDH 36–7
    universalism 37–40
International Classification of Impairments, Disabilities and Handicaps (ICIDH) 9–19
    criticisms 13–19
    cf. ICF 36–7
    Nordenfelt, Prof. Lennart 25–8

judging lives 79, 93
just societies 85–6
justice principle, discrimination 38–40

legal issues
    congenital conditions 8
    Human Fertilisation and Embryology Act (1990) 111
length of life, *good human life* concept 60–2
Lesch–Nyhan syndrome 47–8
Loach, Emma 54–9, 63–4, 72–7, 81–4, 93–4

maximising approach
    challenge 91–4
    critique 87–94
    disabling traits 88–91
    Down's syndrome 67–8, 89
    good human life concept 67–8
    rejecting 93

Maxwell, Robert 79, 122
ME (myalgic encephalomyelitis),
    emergentism 109
medicalisation of disability 15–16, 44,
    46–7
memory functions 14
mental impairment 14
Muhammad Ali 99
moral space 135
moral status 8–9
Morris, Jenny 130
multiple sclerosis (MS) 47–8, 131–4
    emergentism 108–9
Murphy, RF 46
myalgic encephalomyelitis (ME),
    emergentism 109

narrative identity
    disablement 119–23, 137
    Down's syndrome 137
nature of persons, philosophical theories
    98–110
Nordenfelt, Prof. Lennart
    ICIDH 25–8
    theory of disablement 22–5, 28–9,
        41–3
Nozickian view 85–6

objective goods theory
    Down's syndrome 81–4, 90–1
    good human life concept 76–7,
        77–94
ontological individualism 100–4

pain, physicalism 105–6
paradox, defining disablement 5–6
participation restrictions 34–6
    defining 34
permanent vegetative state (PVS) 80,
    112–13
personal existence
    embodiment 126–8
    self-conception 128
    self-project 128–30
    space 124–5
    structuring concepts 123–30

time 125–6
personal identity, disablement 97–110,
    113–19, 119–23
persons
    and human beings 109
    nature of, philosophical theories
        98–110
PGD (prenatal genetic diagnosis) 52,
    97–8, 139
philosophical theories
    dualism 98–104
    emergentism 98, 106–10
    nature of persons 98–110
    physicalism 98, 104–6
physicalism, philosophical theory 98,
    104–6
poverty 8
preference satisfaction as the good life
    deafness 70
    Down's syndrome 69, 72–7
    good human life concept 68–77
    hearing-related preferences 70
    intellectual disabilities 71–2, 90
    sensory disabilities 68–71, 89–90
    syndrome Z 69
pregnancy
    prenatal screening 7–8, 49, 51–2,
        111–12, 141
    terminating 8, 9, 53–9, 111–12
prenatal genetic diagnosis (PGD) 52,
    97–8, 139
prenatal screening 7–8, 49, 51–2,
    111–12, 141
Pride Against Prejudice 130
public/domestic spheres, *good human life*
    concept 65–6
public support 85–6
PVS (permanent vegetative state) 80,
    112–13

racism 38–40
Rawlsian view 85–6
relational concept, disablement 7

screening, prenatal 7–8, 49, 51–2,
    111–12, 141

self-conception, personal existence 128
self-interested concern 116–17
self-project, personal existence 128–30
sensory disabilities
    emergentism 107–8
    preference satisfaction theory 68–71,
       89–90
sensory experiences 92–3
sexism 38–40
Singer, Peter 88, 91
social benefits 8
'social model' of disablement 5–6
space, personal existence 124–5
spinal muscular atrophy 84–5
status, moral 8–9
stomach ulcer 11, 12
structuring concepts
    disablement 130–8
    personal existence 123–30
syndrome Z 53–9, 60
    emergentism 107
    preference satisfaction theory 69

taxation 85
temperature, seeing 92
theory of disablement, Nordenfelt's
    22–5, 28–9, 41–3
threshold approach, *good human life*
    concept 87–8
time, personal existence 125–6

ulcer, stomach 11, 12
Union of the Physically Impaired
    Against Segregation (UPIAS)
    19–22

value laden concept, disablement 7
visual impairment 11, 12, 35
    David Blunkett 45
    justice principle 39

World Health Organization (WHO)
    ICF 32–40
    ICIDH 9–19
    theory of disablement clash 41–3